perspectives in nursing—
1985–1987
based on presentations at the
seventeenth nln biennial convention

wy
16
p467
1985

Pub. No. 41-1985

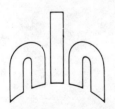

national league for nursing · new york, new york

The views expressed in this publication represent the
views of the authors and do not necessarily reflect the
official views of the National League for Nursing.

Printed in the United States of America

contents

ROLE

QUALITY AND ETHICS

foreword

For those of us fortunate enough to be present at the 17th biennial NLN convention in San Antonio, Texas (June 2–5, 1985), the convention's theme, "Nursing—A Kaleidoscope: Themes and Images for the Future," truly captures the spirit of the event. The papers in this volume, too, attempt to capture the excitement of the original presentations. The scope and depth of these papers, which range from the global to the specific, is proof of the new vitality of nursing as it branches out and reaches into the future.

We were honored to have with us two distinguished speakers opening and closing the convention as they open and close this book. Rollo May and Maggie Kuhn have indeed each presented us with themes and images that can help guide nursing's perspective on the future in these next two years.

Within the kaleidoscope of ideas presented at the convention, the program sessions followed the four main themes that also structure this book: technology; role; quality and ethics; and political and economic aspects of nursing. These themes represent some of the primary preoccupations of nursing now, and probably for some years to come.

Trends in the health care industry and the technology being developed in the society at large affect the way we will teach and practice nursing. The papers in the first section examine the trends to show how we can use technology to help us in education and practice, in research, and in communicating our findings. The next group of papers looks at current problems and suggests ways of mobilizing nurses in all our different roles to address these problems in the future.

In looking to the future, we must also look for ways to assure the continuing quality of nursing service, starting with nursing education that addresses the real needs of society for nurses and health care. Many of these papers analyze the direction of health care today in an attempt to predict these future needs in the various segments of nursing. Finally, in these times of shifting priorities in health care and increasing demands on the health care provider, it is imperative for nursing to find ways to have an impact on the decisions that will, in turn, affect the profession. Papers in this final section show how nurses can work at every level to determine the future of health care and the future of the profession.

Clearly, *Perspectives in Nursing—1985–1987* is truly a forward-looking book. In that sense, it represents the state of the profession in 1985. With this kaleidoscope of ideas to give us perspective, we look forward to 1987 and beyond.

Duane D. Walker
Chairperson
Convention Advisory Committee
Seventeenth Biennial Convention

themes and images
for the future

THE WOUNDED HEALER

ROLLO MAY, PhD

Supervisory and Training Analyst
William Alanson White Institute of Psychoanalysis
Tiburon, California

I take the text for my remarks from the poet T. S. Eliot in his *Four Quartets*. He writes:

> Our only health is the disease.
> If we obey the dying nurse
> Whose constant care is not to please
> But to remind of our, and Adam's curse,
> And that, to be restored, our sickness must grow worse.[1]

Now what did Eliot mean by this?

VIEW OF HEALTH IN SOCIETY

The view of health in our society that is held by the great majority of Americans is that an ailment is simple bad luck. A disease is irrevocable fate. As I have written elsewhere:

> We "fall" ill as though the process were as fateful as gravity. We "catch" a germ as though it were an accident. We are the "victims"

---

[1] From "East Coker," in *Four Quartets*, by T. S. Eliot, copyright 1943 by T. S. Eliot; renewed 1971 by Esme Valerie Eliot. Reprinted by permission of Harcourt Brace Jovanovich, Inc.

of cancer. We "get" sick (instead of "sicken"). And all we can do is be "patient" while the doctor treats us. All these words and phrases are in the passive voice. We assume that we are under the command of some fate and we can do nothing about it. The good patient is considered docile and cooperative, one who puts himself completely in the hands of the physician.[2]

Our conscious selves stand as though we were slaves on the trading block, while other people exercise forces greater than ours.

When I was a young man I had tuberculosis. That was before there were any drugs for the disease, and for several years it was nip and tuck whether I would live or I would die. I had a cavity in my heart about the size of a quarter, and the odds were not great that I could live. I remember for two years simply lying on a bed looking up at the design on the boards in the walls and the ceiling of the room. For the first couple of months, I vowed that I would do exactly what my doctors told me and in this way would hope to get well. But after these two months I discovered I actually was getting worse. And then it occurred to me: Where was my responsibility in this disease? I was the one who picked it up in the first place, and I was the one who now had it within my own body. The doctors readily admitted that they knew very little about tuberculosis. I realized that they were not the ones who had the tuberculosis within them—I was; and until I could take responsibility for this fact, I would continue to get worse. I resolved then that I was the one who had to know the self that I am and to know when I was fatigued, when I was to rest, and when I had the strength and need to exercise.

The important point is that all of these words that we use about illness and disease are in the passive voice. We don't do anything except be patient. This word *patient* is the most telling word of all. I propose that we need in this country a radically different view of health and illness. There are some who agree with me on that point. Dr. Eli Ginzberg, for example, says that "no improvement in the health care system will be efficacious unless the citizen assumes responsibility for his own well-being." And Dr. René Dubos agrees. He says, "Recovery depends upon the mobilization of the patient's own mechanisms of resistance to disease." The problem facing all of us who live in this culture is how we can shift our attitude to the fact that the responsibility is within us rather than simply our being patient or falling ill.

What is the goal and the purpose of health? The ideal of making people healthier and healthier is not adequate. The ideal of living longer and longer is not adequate either. Beyond a certain point, I don't want to live longer. The greater number of people living these days is due most of

---

[2] Rollo May, *Freedom and Destiny* (New York: W. W. Norton & Co., 1981), 204.

all to the lack of infant mortality and not to our advanced inventions. A world that was perfectly healthy would be a completely boring world. The philosopher and Roman emperor Hadrian said way back in the second century, "we know nothing at all about illness so long as we have not recognized its odd resemblance to war and to love, its compromises, its feints, its exactions, that strange and unique amalgam, the mixture of which is produced by a mixture of temperament and a malady." Hadrian is saying that disease and illness are something quite different from what we are taught in our society. It is a strange amalgam between a disease and the temperament that the person has.

How did this wrong idea of health get started? I think we have to look quite seriously at our Faustian world. We notice that on our television sets everbody is smiling and happy, as though life ought to be this jolly affair where one hums one's way through, with a lot of hostility and sex en route. Our whole culture is in the passive voice. Just as Faust had his Mephistopheles who performed magic for him, so we also have our combination of materialism and magic: the magic of money, the magic of gambling, the magic of lottery. In every mail I get three or four letters, sent to everybody, that have big printing on the outside: "Get $1 million." "Join our lottery." "There are $2 million inside this letter for you." Now obviously, there's nothing in there except an advertisement for something. I was brought up to believe that gambling is evil. But in the states that have lotteries it is unpatriotic not to gamble. Every night on television there comes on some man who is groomed to look very respectable, very dependable, who holds out his arms and begs us not to say no to his lottery. "I have 10 million dollars for you," he says, "ten million dollars with your name on it, and I will give it to you in person—ten million dollars just for you."

All of this is utterly evil, because what it does is to lead us into the idea that we all live passively and things are given to us. It is like the bread and circuses that accompanied the fall of ancient Rome. All we have to do is send in this coupon and then we will get a million dollars. This goes hand in hand with the vast number of suicides in our society. The suicide rate for young people is growing rapidly. The reason is not complicated. It is that our society does not challenge them. It gives them hope of always making more money, of getting jobs that will pay more. We have taken away the humanities. They don't learn about the things that give joy. They learn computers, they learn lotteries, they learn all sorts of things that are valuable only because later on they will make money. Young people, who are not yet hardened, need something to love, need some poetry to love, some art to love, something to idealize, something to build their lives around—but this we do not give them. What we give them instead is a culture that builds more and more machines to make more and more money to become richer and richer and leaves out the very soul of human experience. So we no longer live with zest and cannot even die with dignity. It is not surprising that so many young people take to drugs. They take to drugs to fill the great vacuum that comes out of a passive culture, out of the passive view of disease, of work, and of life.

THE WOUNDED HEALER

The notion of the "wounded healer" is the idea that nurses, and that all of us, contribute to other people and to ourselves by virtue of our own wounds. We heal each other, we heal other people, by virtue of our own wounds. It is by virtue of our own wounds that we write poetry, that we paint, that we have compassion and empathy for sick people.

A drama was written about the wounded healer many centuries ago by Sophocles in ancient Greece. *Philoctetes* was written when Sophocles was between the ages of 80 and 90, so we can believe that his greatest wisdom is presented in it. Philoctetes is a Greek warrior going with the other Greeks to fight the Trojan War. This expedition stopped on an island in the Mediterranean to pay homage to the gods. At the shrine, Philoctetes was bitten in the leg by a snake. When they got back on the boat, the wound festered and Philoctetes was in great pain; the other soldiers could not stand the odor or his groans. Odysseus, the clever Greek, proposed that they leave Philoctetes on the next uninhabited island and then go on to Troy. Philoctetes fortunately had a bow, the arrows of which would hit anything it was aimed at. He lived on the island alone, an exile from the Greeks. The Greeks went on to Troy, and for eight years at its walls they made no progress in taking the city. Then a prophet told them that they could never take Troy until they brought Philoctetes back again into the army. So the Greeks dispatched Odysseus, the clever, crafty Greek, with a young man, a boy of 16 or 17, who was the son of Achilles, back to the island to persuade Philoctetes to join the army again.

The drama opens with this boy, Neoptolemus, talking with Odysseus on the shores of the island. Neoptolemus asks Odysseus, "What is virtue?" Neoptolemus answers his own question: "What I think virtue is," he says, "is to tell the truth, to always be on the outside what you are on the inside." And Odysseus, the clever one—who could fit into many of our modern situations—shakes his head and says, "No, virtue is to lie for your country, and after that you have plenty of time to be honest." It is very much what we hear in our day—"My country right or wrong." Finally, Neoptolemus agrees that he will lie for his country and try to persuade Philoctetes. Odysseus hides behind a rock, as Philoctetes comes wandering over the path with his cane and his bow. Neoptolemus talks to him and tells him that he, Neoptolemus, is also angry with the Greeks, that they had betrayed him. He does this as stealth, to persuade Philoctetes that he is the warrior's friend. Philoctetes at first doesn't believe him, but then he does. As they talk together, Philoctetes suddenly has a seizure with the great ulcer on his leg. As Homer puts it, the black red blood flows out. Philoctetes is in agony, and hands his bow to Neoptolemus as he writhes on the ground.

Odysseus knows that once they have the bow, Philoctetes will have to come with them. So he steps out from behind the rock and holds out his hand, saying to Neoptolemus "Give me the bow." But Neoptolemus says "no." He has gone back to his own view of virtue, that virtue is integrity, and is moved to compassion by the suffering of Philoctetes who is lying there on the ground crying to the gods, to please let him die because he is in so much pain. He is empathic with his suffering and he goes back to his own virtue and refuses to take part in this nefarious scheme. It turns out that a message comes from the gods that Philoctetes must go back with the Greeks and his leg will be healed when he gets to Troy.

The meaning of that drama, written some 2,200 years ago, is that through suffering there comes not only empathy, compassion, and sympathy for the suffering one, but there also comes healing. When Philoctetes goes back to Troy he thereupon becomes healed. The wounded man is the hero of that drama, and the healing occurs by virtue of going through his suffering to a more positive and constructive end.

THE PURPOSE OF ILLNESS

What does this mean with respect to our modern day and the profession of nursing? Many very wise modern people as well as people down through the ages have seen the truth as Hadrian saw it—as most of us in our age have not seen it—that, as Nietszche wrote, "strength is restored by wounding." Edmund Wilson, a modern writer, says in his book about Philoctetes, *The Wound and the Bow,* "Superior strength is inseparable from disability." This is why so many creative people who have experienced disease have found that through their *disease* they can give *ease* to other people. Beethoven, through his deafness, through his continuous illness, was able to create beautiful music. The same with Mozart, the same with Chopin, and so many others. There is health in the right attitude toward our disease.

It says in the Bible, "He heals others, himself he cannot heal." There is much more truth in that than most of us realize. The purpose of illness is not simply negation, not simply to get the person up on his feet again. The purpose of illness is to teach us our relationship to nature. One of the old myths in Greece that is perpetually true is about Hercules wrestling with Antaeus. Every time Hercules threw Antaeus to the ground, Antaeus got up again twice as strong. Then Hercules discovered that the earth was the mother of Antaeus and the only way he could win this wrestling match was to hold Antaeus up in the air. The function of disease, the function of illness, is to relate us to our mother, to relate us to nature, to keep us from the arrogance of getting ten million dollars and thinking that this is happiness. That is exactly what destroys our society.

So many creative people down through the ages have experienced severe illness. A British doctor, George Pickering, gathered this data together in a book entitled *Creative Malady.* The subtitle is *Illness in the Lives and Minds of Charles Darwin, Florence Nightingale, Mary Baker Eddy, Sigmund Freud, Marcel Proust and Elizabeth Barrett Browning.* He could have gone on and on, for practically all the creative people down through the ages have created by virtue of their struggle with various forms of ailments and disease. Out of this, says Pickering, come their creative possibilities.

When I had tuberculosis, one of my doctors had on his library shelf a book called *Tuberculosis and Genius.* I borrowed the book—it looked very comforting. It was about all the geniuses down through history who had tuberculosis. The author, a physician, argued that there was some-thing emitted by the bacilli in the body of the sufferer that made that person a genius. This seems to me a stupid reason. Obviously, the ge-niuses worked themselves to pieces, like Mozart did, and whatever they picked up in the way of ailment or illness came by virtue of overwork and not taking care of themselves. This is simply part of the inability to relate their spirit to nature.

Nature is our source, and ultimately we go back to nature when we die. Out of this dialectical relationship between nature and spirit, there comes our genius and our creativity. In *Time* magazine there was an article by K. Jarenson. She studied 47 modern writers and painters, and 18 of them—38 percent—had been hospitalized or treated with lithium or electric shock. The average percentage in our society is 6 percent. What does it mean that six times as many of these talented people have psychiatric ailments for which they give lithium or hospitalize people? Again, it is because the illness, the disease, has something constructive about it. Out of the struggle with disease, with ailment, with illness, there comes a capacity to sense more deeply one's own sensitivity, to sense more deeply what other people are suffering, to understand more pro-foundly, as Hadrian put it, the meaning of illness. Jarenson studied Han-del, Byron, Anne Sexton, Virginia Woolf, and Robert Lowell—possibly the best of modern poets, who was in and out of hospitals. All of these people were manic depressives. But out of Handel came beautiful music, and out of Virginia Woolf and Byron and Robert Lowell came beautiful poetry.

Again we have to ask, What is virtue, what is the value, what is the constructive approach? We can understand from our own illnesses what is the constructive way of using them. We are helped by a study of the people in the concentration camps during the last war—the survivors of Auschwitz and the other concentration camps in Germany. A student, who was a survivor of the concentration camps, wrote a doctoral dissertation pointing out that individuals who have suffered calamitous events in the past can and do function later, not only at average levels, but at even higher than average levels. She writes that "an unusually high number functioned and developed better after the experiences"—either in spite of the calamitous experience or because of it. It may be that the calamitous experience reaches down within us and forces us to find within ourselves greater talent—talent to bear the calamity of the concentration camp, talent to sense beautiful music, talent to help others to paint.

The student also wrote in her dissertation, "The inmates who had had poor, unpampered childhoods adapted best to concentration camps, whereas most of those who had been reared by permissive, wealthy parents were the first to die." This is tremendously interesting, because this is what our young people sense in some inchoate way—that our permissiveness, our wealth, our seductive belief that the richer we get the better off we are, our sense of the richness of our country—these things, they know instinctively, throw them off the track and will lead them not to a happy and productive life, but to a valueless, passive life, to a life in which the deeper values of life are not known.

Illness can operate like an altered state of consciousness. In pain, the "me" is separated from the "not me," and petty ego concerns lose their own pettiness. They become transcended. There is a positive value in being able to feel pain. As Plato said centuries ago, if we could not feel pain we could not also feel pleasure, and the two always go together. Not only do we care for others through our own wounds, but our own wounds may deepen our experience of nature and our experience of our freedom. There is a value in surrendering to forces greater than ourselves.

A dear friend of mine, who is a very good painter, was an alcoholic. He used to drink a pint of vodka a day. He would paint while he was drinking, drink while he was painting—paint all night long. I told him several different times, "Look, you just can't keep this up." Well, he couldn't, and finally he fell into dismay and pleaded with his wife to help him. So she took him to a hospital where he was dehydrated, and then he joined Alcoholics Anonymous. He goes every night. He cannot bear one day to go by without going to an AA meeting. He took me to an AA meeting with him. In this meeting, each one of these persons got up and said, "I am John Jones, an alcoholic. I have been sober for 16 years." Each one calls himself or herself an alcoholic. This is the frankness, the modesty, the exact opposite to the conceit, "Oh what a healthy person I am." They all recognize some power greater than themselves. You can call it nature, you can call it the Absolute, you can call it God, but whatever we posit, whatever words we use, we recognize our ultimate humility, our ultimate feeling, our ultimate conviction that there are powers in the world greater than ourselves. Out of this comes the sense of humility that goes along with the cure. C. G. Jung, the great psychoanalyst, said, "The gods return in our diseases."

BETWEEN HEAVEN AND EARTH

What was the meaning of the last part of the poem from T. S. Eliot? He said: ". . . the dying nurse / Whose constant care is not to please / But to remind of our, and Adam's curse, / And that, to be restored, our sickness must grow worse." Adam's curse stands for the fact that we all are strung between the finiteness of the earth, between nature and the infinity of our imaginations, our beliefs, our yearning for what the alcoholics call a higher power. Again, we see that the function of illness, as T. S. Eliot puts it, is to become aware of the fact that we are finite—we walk around on the earth that is sometimes muddy, sometimes rainy, almost always difficult—but at the same time we have imaginations, and we can use our imaginations to reach beyond our day-to-day existence, to reach beyond our illnesses. Even while we have tuberculosis or something equally severe—even if we have one of the new illnesses that spring up all about us—out of our wounds we will find our creativity and our compassion. Out of this will come our capacity to confront this despair and illness. As Shakespeare put it in *As You Like It,* "Sweet are the uses of adversity, which like the toad, ugly and venemous, yet wears a precious jewel upon its head."

When I think of compassion, there comes to mind the figure back in Springfield, Illinois—a boy who had a terribly difficult life, whose mother died when he was nine, whose father was a ne'er-do-well, a boy who would walk miles and miles to borrow a book to read. This Abraham Lincoln developed a power out of the depths of his own compassion. If he had been alive today he would have been chucked into a hospital, stuffed with lithium in a hurry, and we would have lost perhaps our greatest president. He was depressed, but out of the depression came tremendous compassion, not only for his own self and his own North, but also for the South. Imagine Ronald Reagan saying "let us bind up the wounds of Russia." All of this talk which comes out of Washington as though everybody down there knew what the will of God was and it was very simple—God is what we Americans happen to believe at a given moment. On the contrary, Abraham Lincoln said that a prolongation of the war may be a punishment for the evil of slavery, and he added something that is very refreshing to our souls: "We do not know the purposes of God," he said, "but we know that his judgments are true and righteous altogether." This man could say, "let us live with malice toward none and charity toward all."

We need to understand illness and disability and disease, again, as ways in which our lives remind us that we are finite—we live in the earth where we work, where we hole, where we dig, where we work at often difficult tasks—but we also have imaginations, we have spirits. The fact that we are stretched between heaven and earth is the meaning of human life. Though we walk on earth, we then are in touch with great poetry, great music. Out of our calamities can come our own sensitivity and our own compassion and our own creativity. This is what it means to be a wounded healer.

technology

HEALTH CARE TECHNOLOGY AND THE CHANGING HEALTH CARE SYSTEM

ROGER C. HERDMAN, MD
Assistant Director
Office of Technology Assessment
Congress of the United States
Washington, D. C.

In attempting to illuminate the topic of health care technology and to draw inferences for the nursing profession, I hope that the perspective of one who has worked with the health care system but does not claim in-depth knowledge of nursing practice or education will be useful. This paper is organized into three sections: first, overall trends in mechanization of health care; second, regulatory, financing, and structural changes and their impact; and finally, implications for nursing.

MECHANIZATION OF HEALTH CARE

Those who like to characterize the world with a few catchy words or phrases can describe the evolution of health care over the last few decades as monetarization, corporatization, and mechanization. Monetarization of course refers to the virtual disappearance of charity and philanthropy. Payment systems have developed that assign fees, codes, and reimbursement or prices to every encounter. Philanthropy has shrunk to an insignificant percentage of total support. Corporatization refers to more recent trends: providers organizing in groups of increasing size, corporations managing or providing their own health care, and major for-profit entities taking an increasing share of the health care "business" or in-

15

dustry. Mechanization, to some extent is supported by or results from the other trends, in addition to enjoying increased governmental support for research and development. Mechanization, needless to say, refers to the subject at hand—technology. How much of a role has nursing had and how has it adapted to these three trends?

Mechanization or technology is defined as drugs, devices, and medical care and the organizations and supportive systems within which such care is provided. Intuitively, those in health care sense the extent to which technology as so defined has assumed an ever-expanding importance. There are, however, both direct and indirect data to support this intuition. Direct support comes from examination of the value of sales of devices to health providers. The value of shipments from the device industry has soared from $2 billion to $15 or $16 billion since the passage of Medicare and Medicaid. These figures are impressive, but they relate only to devices and, as noted, technology is much broader than this.

Review of overall resources consumed by the most technologically intensive sectors of the health care system—hospitals and physicians—is a useful indirect measure for estimating the magnitude of the technology factor. Hospitals and physicians, respectively, account for 42 percent and 19 percent of total health care costs; together, they are responsible for just over 60 percent of resources committed to health care. The indirect measures of the effect of technology on these hospital and physician costs are the so-called intensity or residual factors. Overall health system costs have been increasing at rates significantly greater than general inflation for years and have now reached $384 billion a year, or roughly 11 percent of the Gross National Product. Increases in hospital costs have contributed strongly to the overall inflationary trend in health care. For a fairly typical recent year, 59 percent of the increase can be attributed to general inflation; 12 percent to inflation particular to the health sector; and 8 percent to volume increases. The remaining 21 percent of the increase—the residual factor—is assigned to increased intensity of treatment as a result of technology.

Whether inflation is measured per patient day, per admission, or per capita, regardless of the interval chosen, hospital costs are increasing 10 to 17 percent each year. The intensity or technology factor—that is, the quantity of inputs that goes into producing a given unit of hospital care—constitutes 20 to 50 percent of this increase. In the five years before diagnosis related groups (DRGs) were instituted, we found 14 percent per capita inflation, with 40 percent of this inflation due to intensity of service, or technology.[1]

---

[1] Office of Technological Assessment, U.S. Congress, "Medical Technology and Costs of the Medicare Program," OTA-H-227 (Washington, D.C.: U.S. Government Printing Office, July 1984).

In the meantime, the bill for physicians over the last ten years has been growing by about 40 percent more than general inflation. During this time, less technology-oriented primary care physicians have decreased from 44 percent to 39 percent of total physicians, procedural codes have tripled in number, surgical income is up 50 percent more than primary care income, and surgical rates are up 22 percent an hour. An hour of hospital care is twice as costly and an hour of surgical care five times as costly as an office visit hour.

Data from the Medicare program show that while fee increases contributed from 6 to 10 percent of increasing physician payments each year, the total payment increases have been one-and-a-half times and, more recently, twice this amount.[2] This increasing difference between fee increase and total increase—the so-called residual after fee changes are accounted for—is ascribed to more and higher-cost services and use of technology.

The conclusion is that American medicine is becoming more technologically oriented. The questions are, what are nurses doing about this, and what effects will recent changes in payments and adjustments to this trend have on the technological imperative?

CHANGES IN THE SYSTEM

Recent changes in the health care system have included (1) a new emphasis on technology assessment by government and other payers, hospitals (both profit and nonprofit) and industry; (2) the effects of changes in financing that alter incentives and may alter the total resources available to hospitals and laboratories, as well as the possible effects of threatened changes in physician reimbursement; and (3) changes in the sites and management of services.

Emphasis on Technology

Traditionally, technologies have been introduced in health care with either little or no official examination or only a review of safety. The Food and Drug Administration was concerned about safety of drugs, and the medical establishment, on occasion and in a minority of instances, carried out clinical trials for new procedures. A combination of circumstances over the last several decades has led to several major changes in this historical practice, however. Among these have been the extension of regulation to devices; the addition of examination for effectiveness for their labeled uses of technologies such as drugs and devices; the current

---

[2] Special Committee on Aging, "Medicare: Paying the Physician—History, Issues and Options," information paper, 98th Congress, 2nd Sess. (Washington, D.C.: U.S. Government Printing Office, 1984).

interest of government, providers (both profit and nonprofit), industry, and third-party payers in expanded technology assessment; and the development and emphasis on technology assessment itself as a tool, not just for evaluating safety and efficacy for intended use, but as a way of determining cost-effectiveness and social and ethical implications of new and existing technologies.

These changes, such as the addition of review of effectiveness and devices to the Federal Food, Drug and Cosmetic Act, reflect legitimate concerns that technologies be able to accomplish the effects intended and promised by their developers and marketers. But just as important and more relevant to this discussion has been the recent emphasis on a broader examination of technologies. This new concern presupposes that safety and efficacy are no longer enough. In an atmosphere of cost containment and close reexamination of the overall benefits of our health system, we also need to examine whether a technology has sufficient advantages to justify its cost and to explore its broad social and ethical implications for our system of health care.

This need for more intensive scrutiny was pointed out in the late 1960s by the National Academy of Sciences and was also recognized by Congress at about that time. The development and use of a technology was not justified, according to this line of thinking, simply because it was possible. For example, the costs might be disproportionate and lead to a trade-off in which other more useful interventions were foregone because resources were limited. Discussions of the artificial heart often exemplify this line of thought.

A number of institutions are involved for various purposes in this expanded assessment of technology. The Congressional Office of Technology Assessment began its work in the early 1970s by pioneering the development of methodologies for health technology assessment and has continued with a number of general and specific studies. More recently, the Office of Health Care Technology Assessment of the National Center for Health Services Research, which is responsible for recommending coverage by Medicare, has begun to consider broadening its scope of work from more classical considerations of safety and efficacy. The Institute of Medicine has a new mandate to enter this field in a comprehensive way, but to date has not done so.

State governments also have become involved in managing technology. For example, New York State, often the leader in innovations in the health field, has recently created a joint academic-state organization, the New York State Center for Assessing Health Services, to gather information on health care technology and to initiate statewide discussions with all concerned parties, including providers, legislators, and payers. Thus, at all levels, national, state, and local, as the discussion that follows indicates, technology is recognized as a subject that deserves close scrutiny by all those involved with its development and use.

Changes in Health Care Financing

Of particular interest among the changes affecting the health care system has been the response of an array of institutions to the incentives and financial pressures posed by Medicare's new prospective payment (DRG) system for hospitals. Although nurses are currently underrepresented in these responses, they have a lot to contribute, and not just from the nursing perspective of caring, of attending to the whole patient, of interest in health education, of delivering certain kinds of services. Nurses' contribution may derive as well from intimate knowledge that stems from these perspectives—knowledge that is refined by the practical considerations of being on the scene and using and observing the technologies 24 hours a day. Perhaps nurses need to pay more attention in education and in professional practice to technologies. In this discussion of technology and specific institutional responses, nurses may identify ways to increase their involvement.

The institutions responding to the new financial situation include businesses that are self-insuring and third-party payers, both of which are making cost-effectiveness decisions as to which technologies they will cover. Hospitals themselves are reviewing acquisitions differently and with greater care. In many cases, hospitals are no longer buying technologies or instituting procedures and services just because physicians ask for them. They are making business decisions based on whether technologies will pay back their costs in short periods of time or will have positive marketing implications. They are seeking single vendors, discounts, new markets, and new joint ventures. Manufacturers of health products are responding by developing and marketing on a cost-effectiveness basis.

The DRG system is complex in its incentives, as some examples will show, but the implications for diffusion of technologies are so significant that Congress established an important commission, the Prospective Payment Assessment Commission (ProPAC), to look at and recommend responses to the diffusion of new technology. Congress has recently recognized the urgency of having nursing representation on the commission, and legislation has been introduced to expand the commission to enable the appointment of a professional nurse. Nurses are already participating most usefully at the staff level in ProPAC.

This is a difficult arena. Evaluations that balance potential benefits and health outcomes against risks and costs may be tricky and are often subjective. However, the added dimension of the multiple, sometimes conflicting, financial aspects of the DRG system and the decisions regarding changing it to accommodate new technologies create even more problems for technology assessment.

A few examples will help to illustrate these difficulties. The extracorporeal shock wave lithotripter (the noninvasive fragmentation of kidney stones by shock waves) raises issues of coding. Since there is no procedural code currently, whether this procedure will be assigned to a surgical or medical DRG is uncertain, but the decision will have major implications for reimbursement. Substitution of a noninvasive procedure for major surgery, which could cut hospital stay at least in half, also has major benefits for both patient care and cost. As long as capital costs (about $2 million in this case) are reimbursed completely and separately and DRG prices apply only to operational costs, operating savings will favor this technology. Modification of the capital payment system is likely soon, however. These issues of coding, DRG assignment, and capital will enter into decisions about whether to acquire and use what may be a quality-enhancing, cost-reducing technology and whether to locate it under inpatient, outpatient, or freestanding auspices.

Percutaneous transluminal coronary angioplasty currently is assigned to the coronary bypass surgery DRG. This technology uses an expandable catheter to mechanically open atherosclerotic coronaries; under even the most pessimistic scenarios it is 15 percent cheaper than bypass surgery. If it fails, as it often does, a bypass can still be performed. The incentives here encourage hospital acquisition and use—in fact, perhaps even overuse—of the technology. However, ProPAC has recommended assigning angioplasty to a medical DRG with a much reduced price. Even under present conditions, angioplasty followed by bypass is a money-maker only if bypass is performed for a separate payment during a separate admission. Changing DRGs or policing second admissions can drastically alter incentives to use such a procedure.

Implantable infusion pumps appear to have a lot to offer patients receiving cancer chemotherapy. Their costs are considerable, however, and because they are a new technology, the costs are not adequately reflected in most cancer DRGs. DRG incentives to minimize costs may well discourage use of this technology, even though in the long run better therapy may decrease complications and subsequent hospitalizations, producing a total cost savings and health benefit.

The same logic applies, to some extent, to intraocular lens implantation, which enhances quality and increases cost. In this case, the twist is that without an additional allocation for this procedure in the DRG (which ProPAC has recommended against for the time being) the procedure can and will be moved to the outpatient or even nonhospital setting, where costs are reimbursed. If reimbursement for the DRG includes the lens cost, patients may be "Ping Ponged" back to the inpatient setting, necessitating careful monitoring by the peer review organization to ensure that the assigned treatment and site is based on medical necessity rather than financial considerations, and so on.

Thus, as health technology has become more and more important and the system has moved from considerations of safety, to safety and efficacy, to safety, efficacy, and cost-effectiveness and other broader aspects, it has reached the point where complex financial and organizational issues are increasingly influencing decisions that were originally based on considerations of safety, efficacy, and cost-effectiveness. These new influences now appear to have reshaped the historical trends for hospital and technology costs reviewed earlier. However, it is still early to reach conclusions on the shape of new trends.

Reorientation of Services

Because the various sections of the health care system interact with one another so closely, it is important to look at the effects of changes in the system on areas other than the hospital. Changes that will shrink the supply of hospital beds, or at least promote more rapid turnover of patients, also lead to the expansion of long-term care, home health care, and various outpatient and ambulatory settings and affect their emphasis and capacity and the development and application of new technologies in these settings. At the same time, the dramatic aging of the population in the United States will result in continued strong demand for services, especially for chronic conditions. With the development of new technologies for enteral and parenteral nutrition, incontinence, long-term and outpatient therapy, sight and hearing impairment, helping the aged function in the home environment, and self-help programs, nurses will be called upon to understand and use these technologies to design, coordinate and implement the necessary treatment programs.

For the first time, the majority of doctors are no longer individual entrepreneurs but are functioning in organized settings, working in group practices, preferred provider organizations, health maintenance organizations, and independent practice associations and for hospitals and major corporations. Also for the first time, many of these organizations are led by non-physicians, and for the first time there is substantial vertical and horizontal integration and substantial profit-making activity in health care. These factors suggest an environment in which attention to professional concerns will take a back seat to business considerations of profit and loss. Finally, while pressures from cost-conscious or prudent buyers, such as insurers and federal and state governments, may limit the availability of funding and other resources and, as noted, change the scope of growth and the cost curve for the health care system, I nevertheless believe that Congress will make available funding for adequate use of technology and provision of quality care and that private resources will follow. What we are seeing, many predict, is a shakeout that will allow for reestablishment of growth from a somewhat lower base.

IMPLICATIONS FOR NURSING

These widespread changes in the health care system have many implications for the future of nursing. The practice of nursing involves understanding and using technology, just as the practice of physicians does. In many cases, however, nursing services may be more cost-effective than physician services, even in the face of an oversupply of physicians. Many cost-conscious health care organizations could be persuaded that nurses get the job done more efficiently. Nurses who understand new health technologies and grasp the changes and opportunities that result from their use will have an important role in the implementation and evaluation of technology in the broadest sense.

Nurses have traditionally utilized complicated technologies as they have become available in various health care settings. In high-technology settings, such as intensive care units, coronary care units, neonatal intensive care units, and dialysis units, it is nurses who best apply the technologies. Now, however, nurses find themselves in an environment that is rapidly changing and becoming increasingly technological. Hospitals are cutting back on full-time equivalent staff and beginning to look for personnel who are more flexible and cost efficient. At new sites of service, the same standards will apply.

These pressures will affect nursing practice, education, and research. As the number of sites for clinical experience decreases, their quality should increase. Is tomorrow's nurse learning to understand the new technologies and the new environments? Contacts with recent graduates are not reassuring. Many do not understand computers and the tremendous role they are playing in helping patients, in assisting providers with innovative software and diagnostic and treatment algorithms. They do not understand the uses of computers in the high-technology environments such as the intensive care unit. Nor have students, in many cases, reviewed the new home care technologies and the array of assistive technologies for chronic conditions. There must be a place to gain education and experience about what technologies can do for people and how to evaluate them. This would give nurses a greater role in decision making and the flexibility and cost-effectiveness to become even more valuable as central health care providers. Nurses are extremely capable in applying technologies—skills they learn primarily on the job; they should also be educated about the broader values, principles, and roles of technology.

Are nursing organizations taking enough time to think through the current changes and opportunities and talk to corporations and business groups or organized health providers who are interested more in cost-effective quality health outcomes? Are they jointly determining with these groups how nurses can contribute to health care in such settings, where good management and competitive quality care are the major considerations?

In the great majority of primary care and many specialty care situations, well-trained nurses or specially trained nurse practitioners should be highly competitive. They are cost-effective, achieve good performance levels, generate good patient satisfaction and increased compliance, improve patient education, and result in fewer returns and hospitalizations when properly utilized. In such situations, where the issue is organized buyer satisfaction, not physician satisfaction, surpluses of physicians become irrelevant. Nurses need to discover such niches, ensure proper training for them, and market nursing services.

In a technological age, understanding of technologies is part of the preparation and need not impair the other assets for which nurses are valued. It has recently been reported that the nursing evaluation and plan is twice as good a predictor of DRG costs as the medical diagnosis. If this is true, cost-conscious providers would certainly pay attention to nursing technologies, and nurses would find it worth their while to be educated to assume roles of explaining, deciding, managing patients, and coordinating services and technologies.

As nurses become more sophisticated in this area, they should find themselves in a better position to handle the ethical problems, that can only become more pressing as our population ages. Stories appear with increasing frequency in newspapers or on television about controversies over the application of life-sustaining techniques to the seriously or terminally ill, the very old, or the severely handicapped. Questions about the use or misuse of technologies, the understanding of what technologies can do, the rights of patients, and the liabilities and the ethics of these situations are part of a continuing public debate. Nurses seem to be caught up in this debate with neither the opportunity to participate authoritatively (even though they are usually allowed representation on ethics committees) nor the necessary breadth of ethical training and expertise. And yet, often it is the nurse who best knows the patient's wishes, the patient's condition, and the patient's family. A more independent role for nurses in the provision of health care would help, when this can be achieved. Also, better grounding in technology assessment and basic ethics would go a long way toward according nurses a more authoritative role in the debate. In short, nurses should be engaged in a process of developing a professional ethical consensus. If this is being done, it is surely not well known. What one often hears about is disputes between physicians who are reluctant to actually "pull the plug" themselves and nurses who are not in a strong position to debate the issue.

CONCLUSION

My objective in this discussion has been to sketch out the existing and changing features of technology and the health care system and to suggest implications for nursing. It is first necessary to understand technology or mechanization as a major and continuing trend. Then nurses can understand and deal with technology better while preserving their traditional strengths. There are roles for managing and evaluating technology at all levels and for all participants. In addition, proper education can improve nurses' performance and assist them in realizing the opportunities created by change if nurses work together and plan, not necessarily by turning into physicians or supertechnicians, but by enhancing skills and abilities they already have. New payment and organizational environments are opening up possibilities for new roles and emphasizing the strengths and financial importance of nurses and nursing technology. The possibilities are so numerous that with the exercise of skill and foresight, the future looks bright indeed.

HIGH TOUCH IN A HIGH-TECH FUTURE

MARTHA E. ROGERS, ScD, RN, FAAN
Professor Emerita, Division of Nursing
School of Education, Health, Nursing, and Arts Professions
New York University
New York, New York

Adapting for my own use a statement made some years ago, I would say that it is not high technology that is causing our trouble, rather it is the people "whose feet tread the earth of a new world as their heads continue to dwell in the past." [1] Whether "those people" are scientists clinging to outdated world views, proponents of people as machines or collections of chemicals, nurses reluctant to exchange old technical resources for new tools of practice, or those fearful of unemployment generated by accelerating technological diversity—the argument prevails that high technology contradicts humane human services. In nursing, the debate too often sinks to this level of "high touch" versus "high tech," a view that overlooks the importance of both as tools in the knowledgeable practice of the science of nursing from which people may benefit.

---

[1] George S. Counts, "The Impact of Technological Change," in *The Planning of Change*, ed. W. G. Bennis et al. (New York: Holt, Rinehart & Winston, 1962), 21.

'IF THIS IS THE FUTURE . . .'

In December 1963 the Research Institute of America published a bulletin that began:

> The moment of truth on automation is coming . . . a lot sooner than most people realize. . . . The actions taken to cope with the coming crisis of automation will be more radical than business and government leaders publicly admit. . . . Automation has just begun to bite in. Up to now techniques have been in the process of development; today the major systems are complete. From this point on, they'll be spreading rapidly. The effect will be revolutionary on everything from office and plant to society itself.

The nearly 25 years since then have witnessed major developments in automation, rapid shifts in the state of the art in computers, thriving robots, and space travel, with moon villages and space towns soon to be realized.

Futurologists abound, although their predictions do not always match developments in real time. For instance, an article in *Science 84* was titled: "If this is the future—where's my 13 hour work week, personal helicopter, household robot, air-conditioned street, and auto pilot car?" [2] But do not despair. These and other wonders are in process.

When Thomas A. Edison invented the electric light, a demonstration for the public was installed in a New Jersey community. A committee of Englishmen came over to view this wonder and find out if it would really last. More specifically, they wanted to determine if the gas lighters would soon be out of jobs. The committee returned home confident that the electric light would never replace the gaslight. Today not only has the gas lighter passed into history, but it seems likely that the meter-reader may follow, as plans for a high-tech gas meter are implemented. Diversified Energies, parent company of the Minneapolis-based Minnegasco gas company, has applied for a patent on a radio-controlled gas meter that would transmit a signal to a central computer, which would automatically calculate the customer's bill.

A computer in every home is joining the chicken in every pot as the societal ideal. We are pressured to buy, buy, buy for home, school, and workplace on the high-tech market. Twenty years ago Secretary of Labor Willard Wirtz stated: "The machine now has a high school education in the sense that it can do most jobs that a high school graduate can do, so machines will get the job because they work for less than a living wage. A person needs 14 years of education to compete with a machine." [3] Today many fourth and fifth graders are computer literate. In

---

[2] *Science 84* (January 1984): 34–43.

[3] *Time*, March 5, 1965, 60.

less than another decade it can be expected that students entering college may be more comfortable with computers than the previous generation was with typewriters. College campuses are getting powerful new machines that can enhance education and research.

Not only are educational institutions rolling in computers, but the health care industry is alive with them. Nor is this a new event. In 1964, several departments at the Children's Hospital in Akron, Ohio, were linked to a central computer. It was predicted that nurses might have as much as 40 percent more time to spend with patients. Computer systems in hospitals and in a range of health care agencies look after patient records, record and analyze vital signs, collect patient histories, regulate medications, diagnose and treat, analyze test results, monitor vital signs and intravenous transfusions, and so forth, ad infinitum. Last year, *Omni* magazine carried an article about robot nurses.

Machines do *not* provide human services. Nor are machines a substitute for knowledgeable nursing services. Nonetheless, when used wisely and with judgment machines can be useful adjuncts on tools of practice. Their effectiveness and safety require nurses who are knowledgeable in the science of nursing, who are committed to people and their world as the focus of their concern, and who are socially responsible.

High technology is a manifestation of humankind's continuously innovative potential. Nostalgia for the "good old days" should not be allowed to obscure the "good old" outhouses, lack of central heating, and the other inconveniences that accompanied them.

THE JOB FRONTIER

High technology presages a new job frontier. Fear of unemployment as new machines are introduced is not new. That people are affected by accelerating technology is reflected in such phenomenon as attrition without replacement of personnel, layoffs, and retraining programs. But these are by no means all attributable to high technology. Change is inevitable, and it is escalating on many fronts in many ways.

Moreover, one might reasonably propose that in the long term, as in the past, more jobs will be created than destroyed. Already there are mismatches between the nature of the labor supply and the demand for it. Preparing persons for jobs that are obsolete or no longer exist is tragic human waste. The past does not control the future.

"High tech" and "high touch" are not, in themselves, adversaries. Rather, the problem lies with nurses who perceive manual and machine skills as the substance of nursing rather than as tools that may be useful to implement the science of nursing. Many nurses have become enamored of machines. Pervasive anti-educationism, dependency, and naiveté have exacerbated many problems. Concomitantly, the struggle for scientific identity and recognition as a learned profession continue to engage growing numbers of nurses.

"High touch" is a kind of shorthand for personal caring for people. It need not be physical touch, though it may include physical touch. It is a tool of practice. It has significance when it is rooted in a firm foundation in the science of nursing.

Some 25 years ago Elizabeth Kemble, then dean of the School of Nursing at the University of North Carolina at Chapel Hill stated:

> much has been written and said concerning the spirit, art, and science of nursing. No one will deny the importance of all three in the effective practice of nursing. But the noble spirit alone is not enough. The art of nursing falls far short even with a fine spirit. It is only when nursing practice is based on a theoretically sound foundation that the spirit and art can come into full being.[4]

Predicting the future can be dangerous. We live in a probabilistic world. We are also participants in creating the future. This future is by and large already here if we but open our eyes to see.

NURSING TODAY AND TOMORROW

Nursing today is perceived by many to be in a state of crisis. The Chinese write the word *crisis* with two characters: the first signifies *danger* and the second *opportunity*. Nursing evolves within the larger world of people's experience. The health care system is in rapid change. It is up to us to seize the opportunities and to act with courage that people may benefit. Robert Browning's words, "A man's reach should exceed his grasp else what's a heaven for," are worth pondering.

Power, profits, and tradition vie with a "high tech/high touch" future. Cost containment has become a byword as diagnosis related groups (DRGs) seek to put a cap on rampaging overcharges by hospitals and physicians. But the situation is much larger and more complex than DRGs. Community-based health services are growing rapidly. A variety of health workers crowd the marketplace. Nearly 40 percent of nurses do not work in hospitals now. Before long this percentage can be expected to increase to the point where the larger percentage of nurses will work in community-based centers.

In Texas, 21 hospitals filed billions of dollars in false Medicare claims in a scandal that, according to the U.S. General Accounting Office, rivals defense contract overcharges.[5] And it seems unlikely that Texas hospitals

---

[4] Elizabeth Kemble, *Unity of Nursing Care* (Chapel Hill, N.C.: University of North Carolina, June, 1960).

[5] *Dallas Morning News*, June 2, 1985; *USA Today*, June 3, 1985.

are alone in massive Medicare overcharges. Hospitals are big business and big bucks. The second highest paid corporate executive in the United States last year according to *Forbes Magazine* is head of Humana, Inc., at nearly $18 million. Profit-making hospitals seem to be doing well.

The idea of people as machines and collections of spare parts wherewith to robotocize human beings enamors many. Human experimentation is not uncommon, and informed consent seems to have many meanings. A mechanist philosophy contradicts the unitary nature of humankind and our world and emerging world views.

Dislocations in the job market are already being felt in nursing. Blaming all of these on DRGs and other similar events will not solve the problems. We have too many nurses prepared for jobs that are not needed and too few to initiate and fill the jobs in nursing that are needed. Moreover, the practice of nursing focuses on people. Nursing does not exist to serve the ends of any other field. The practice of nursing does not mean learning how to run a computer or how to nurse machines.

What kinds of nurses and practitioners of nursing are needed? How should nurses be prepared so that human health and welfare may be promoted?

Nursing is a learned profession—a science and an art. The term *nursing* is thus a noun signifying a body of abstract knowledge arrived at by scientific research and logical analysis. The science of nursing is a new product: a synthesis of facts and ideas about the phenomenon of our concern. The phenomenon central to nursing identifies the uniqueness of nursing. No other field focuses on human beings as irreducible phenomena integral with their environmental fields.

Principles and theories derive from nursing's conceptual system. They are *not* a collection of principles and theories from other fields. Nursing as a science is not identified by a collection of skills and techniques. Skills and techniques are tools and may indeed enhance the practice of nursing, but they are not nursing knowledge.

Learned professional education in nursing demands a broad foundation in the liberal arts and sciences and substantive knowledge in the theoretical basis of nursing. The National Institute of Education's recent report criticizes the excessively vocational orientation of bachelor's degree programs and states that "all bachelor's degree recipients should have at least two full years of liberal education. In most professional fields, this will require extending undergraduate programs beyond the usual four years." [6] The baccalaureate degree is the first professional degree in nursing and requires five years. General education, both lower- and upper-division, not only includes such subject matter as literature, history,

---

[6] Ezra Bowen, "Bringing Colleges Under Fire," *Time*, October 29, 1984, 78.

mathematics, philosophy, the biological world, the physical world, the social and psychological worlds, politics and government, but also needs to include computer literacy and "extraterrestrial" knowledge. Education in nursing builds on a broad general foundation, is theoretically based in the science of nursing, and is concerned with all people wherever they are. Opportunities to test theoretical learnings are provided in real-world laboratory settings that are predominantly community based, in contrast to the current overemphasis on hospital settings. In fact, any school that emphasizes hospitals as the primary nursing arena will contribute to the nation's unemployed and unemployable in nursing. This is not to propose that no nurses will work in hospitals, but hospitals will not be the primary employer. Health services are vastly more broadly based.

Baccalaureate education is the cornerstone of nursing's educational system. Nursing has long had three entry levels to practice and licenses for only two of these—the practical nurse level and the registered nurse level for which associate degree and hospital schools prepare. There is critical need for an additional license for the baccalaureate level of nursing practice. It is the baccalaureate graduate who is the peer of engineers, medical doctors, dentists, lawyers, social workers, and other professionals. Only those already licensed nurses holding a baccalaureate degree with an upper-division major in nursing that was approved at the time the person graduated would be "grandfathered" in to be automatically entitled to receive the new baccalaureate-level license.

There is also continuing need for registered nurses prepared in associate degree programs. The education of all nurses belongs squarely in and controlled by educational institutions. The historical accident that placed nurse preparation in hospitals is an unfortunate event that should long since have been rectified.

Qualified faculty in nursing are indispensable. The fad of joint appointments only threatens to make us "jacks of all trades and masters of none."

Nursing practice will encompass independent nursing practice, autonomous nursing centers, and autonomous birthing centers, without the fallacy of so-called medical backup. However, standards of practice will be commensurate with educational preparation. Professional responsibility will rest with those holding valid baccalaureate and higher degrees in nursing.

There is critical need for mutual respect for differences among nurses and for differences between nurses and other personnel. Noninvasive modalities will predominate. All of us must undergo continual "retreading" for this new world. As we engage in the job that is before us there will be no time for burnout. We must *get out* of old ruts instead of *cop out* because of failure to envision the future.

An analogy to the situation of nursing today is that of an embryo in its eighth month in utero. It realizes things seem to be getting crowded.

There is lots of waste floating around. The situation looks quite dismal. Then it begins to imagine what it might be like in the ninth month, the tenth, the eleventh month. The vision is truly frightening. What the embryo fails to realize is that in the ninth month there will be a major change—birth.

VIDEO-TELECONFERENCING IN NURSING

FRANCES C. HENDERSON, RN, EdD
Project Coordinator
California Statewide Project for Service-Education
Consensus on Associate Degree Nurse Competency
Ohlone College
Fremont, California

Video-teleconferencing presents nursing with a kaleidoscope of possibilities by which to communicate the themes and images of the future. Video-teleconferencing is an ideal medium for the dissemination of content that would benefit from timely distribution and visual presentation to geographically dispersed audiences of nurses. It is an ideal instructional mode as well, especially if immediate and active participation on the part of the learners is desired.

The advantages of video-teleconferencing far outweigh the one disadvantage of high production costs. These costs can be offset by using any one of a variety of strategies or an optimum combination. Registration fees can be established based on the proportion of the total number of viewers reached to the cost of production. Another strategy is to seek external grant funding in an amount sufficient to cover production costs. Shared sponsorship by vendors whose goods or services can be marketed in printed materials that participants will receive or through creative video media or exhibits in conjunction with the video-teleconference are other viable strategies to offset the high cost of production. An edited videotape and relevant printed materials can also be marketed after the program.

The immediate advantages of video-teleconferencing include the opportunity for a multimedia approach to content delivery through the use of live presentations by experts; live panel or roundtable discussions, and pretaped videographics, vignettes, or documentaries. Live, interactive question-and-answer exchanges may be arranged between content experts at the origination site and audiences in geographically distant locations. Video-teleconferencing also eliminates the necessity for prolonged absence from work and minimizes outlays for travel, lodging, and other expenses associated with participation in conventional one-time, one-place conferences. Among the longer-term benefits of video-teleconferencing is dissemination after the conference of selected portions of the live program through edited videotapes of the proceedings. The audio-track of the videotaped conference may also be translated into other languages for international use.

The key to determining whether or not video-teleconferencing is the medium most suitable to the needs of a particular program is the timeliness and visual nature of the content, the location of the audience, and the potential benefits of active audience participation.

VIDEO-TELECONFERENCING EXPERIENCES

The pioneering efforts of Ohlone College in Fremont, California, in the area of video-teleconferencing began in 1982. With funding by the W. K. Kellogg Foundation of Battle Creek, Michigan, nursing project staff at Ohlone College and Yonchenko-Hecht Media Productions of San Francisco planned and produced their first national video-teleconference, which was aired in June 1983.[1] The purpose of this five-hour conference, "The Ohlone Transition," was twofold. First, the project staff disseminated the outcomes of a preceptorship project in the Associate Degree Program at Ohlone College. Second, the conference served as a pilot test of the medium to determine its potential application as an optimum method of disseminating information. The results were highly favorable. A one-year follow-up study of 544 participants showed that 92 percent of the respondents would attend another videoconference and would recommend this type of conference to their staff.

Building on this initial success, a four-hour California statewide instructional video-teleconference was presented in October 1983 in conjunction with the California Statewide Project for Service-Education Consensus on Associate Degree Nurse Competency. The purposes of this program, "Objective Assessment of Clinical Competence," were to present the underlying concepts of objective assessment of clinical competence and

---

[1] An edited videotape of this program, *The Ohlone Transition*, is available from the American Journal of Nursing Company, New York City.

examples of how the concepts were adapted by one nursing program. The program allowed participants to apply the concepts in simple video-taped simulations. Audiences at 11 sites in California participated in off-the-air discussion just prior to the on-the-air program and in a one-hour practice session immediately after the program. A two-hour edited vid-eotape of the program, with supporting printed materials was made available to those who wanted to improve their clinical evaluation skills but were unable to attend the live program. This method more than doubled the total number of nurses who were able to participate in this learning activity.

In June 1984, the Interproject Network of nursing projects funded by the W. K. Kellogg Foundation, one of which was located at Ohlone College, chose a national nursing video-teleconference as the best method to disseminate the projects' results. A one-year project located at Ohlone College and funded by the W. K. Kellogg Foundation, produced a national nursing video-teleconference, entitled "Associate Degree Nursing: The Intent, the Reality, the Future," scheduled to air on November 7, 1985.

SUCCESSFUL VIDEO-TELECONFERENCING

These successful video-teleconferencing experiences have provided an evolving framework for producing a successful video-teleconference. Collaboration between nursing project staff and Yonchenko-Hecht Media Productions has been the single most crucial factor to the successes of these video-teleconferences. With a collective commitment to excellence, open communication, realistic flexibility, and respect for individual expertise, the nursing project staff and the media consultants collaboratively define roles and responsibilities and work through a systematic and detailed program-planning process for each production. This collaborative planning, implementation, and evaluation process lasts from 9 to 18 months.

To begin, the nursing project staff specify in a planning outline, provided by the media production consultants, the purpose, objectives, content overview, and audience of the conference, as well as the rationale for using a video-teleconference as the medium of choice. Together, nursing project staff and media production consultants explore such questions as:

1. Would the video-teleconferencing medium enhance the desired outcomes specified in the cognitive, psychomotor, and affective objectives?

2. How desirable is it to reach a large number of nurses in geographically distant locations simultaneously?

3. Is an interactive format suitable and desirable for the content?

Early in the planning process, the media production consultants submit a detailed proposal for the production, including a proposed program format, viewing sites, filming schedules, and a budget. Once this proposal is satisfactorily negotiated, program planning progresses with activities such as:

1. Securing the origination site, remote viewing sites, and production crew.
2. Developing a detailed minute-by-minute program format.
3. Selecting and preparing content presenters, site facilitators, and the moderator.
4. Scheduling the day, time, and length of the program.
5. Scripting the entire program.
6. Coordinating program production.
7. Filming video inserts.

Other factors that have contributed to the video-teleconference successes are the selection of content that is relevant to a broad audience of nurses; scheduling of the program to accommodate the majority of the audience to be addressed; and the careful selection of content experts, the program moderator, and a cadre of well-prepared site facilitators statewide and nationwide. Site facilitators play an important role in briefing audiences about the call-in question protocol, issuing packets of materials and continuing education certificates, and guiding group discussion and group participation, as appropriate, at the remote viewing sites. Early, ongoing, and highly active promotion of the program is a must. Other crucial details are arranging the provision of continuing education units, preparing printed materials for participants, and planning and implementing registration. Evaluation forms must be designed that include ratings of the extent to which the content objectives were met and the technical quality of the production. Figure 1 illustrates the ingredients nursing project staff have identified for successful video-teleconferencing.

CONCLUSION

Planning and producing an effective interactive video-teleconference is an exciting, challenging, and perpetually rewarding experience. This medium expands the range of instructional and dissemination modes available to nurses by bringing together the drama, color, and motion of television with interaction via telephone. It provides a highly participatory approach for the sharing of information critical to nursing with large audiences of nurses in geographically distant locations in a cost-effective

Figure 1. Ingredients for a Successful Video-Teleconference

Program Planning
Relevant content
Clear program objectives
Content enhanced by video format
Scripting

Formats
Variety
Well-organized segments

High-Level Interactiveness
Well-informed moderator
Ample question-and-answer segments
Off-air time before and after conference
for audience and facilitators to
interact

Necessary Considerations

Scheduling
Day of week
Time of day
Length—3–4 hours

Viewing Site
Easily accessible
Offering adequate technical
equipment
Environment conducive to learning

**Facilitators and
Technical Experts**
Well prepared
Content expertise
(if required)
Group skills

Audio Contact
Dedicated phone lines
Clear telephone protocol plan
for screening questions

Assurances for Success

Long- and Short-Term Marketing Plan	Registration	Survey of Identified Audience
Identified target groups Variety of advertising methods	Organized by site from central office	Interest in content Geographic location

People Who Make it Happen
(Production Team)

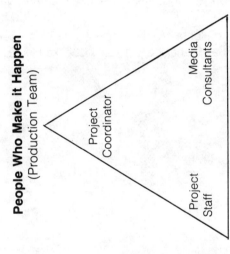

Project
Coordinator

Project
Staff

Media
Consultants

Source: Sharlene Limon, MS, RN, Field Consultant, California Statewide Project for Service-Education Consensus on Associate Degree Competency, Ohlone College, Fremont, California.

manner. In our information-driven, high-technology society, interactive video-teleconferencing expands and enriches nurses' kaleidoscopic view of salient themes and images now and for the future.

BIBLIOGRAPHY

Limon, Sharlene, Judith B. Spencer, and Frances C. Henderson. "Video-Teleconferencing by Nurses—for Nurses." *Nursing & Health Care* 6 (June 1985): 313–317.

Spencer, Judith B., Frances C. Henderson, and Sharlene Limon. "Planning Video-Teleconferences for Nurses in Education and Practice." *Health Care Conference Planner* (July 1984).

Waters, Verle, and Helen Hanson. "Nursing Video-Teleconference Extension Project." Unpublished report. Fremont, Calif.: Ohlone College, July 1984.

Yonchenko-Hecht Media Productions. *Video Teleconferencing Planning Guide.* San Francisco, Calif.: Yonchenko-Hecht Media Productions, 1983.

IMPLEMENTING COMPUTER TECHNOLOGY IN NURSING EDUCATION

CAROL A. ROMANO, RN, MS
Nursing Consultant
Nursing Information System Specialist
Nursing Department, Clinical Center
National Institutes of Health
Bethesda, Maryland

Computer technology continues to be a dominant force in the health care delivery system. Educational preparation in this area equips the nurse to take an active leadership role in the design of computerized systems that affect the delivery of nursing care. In addition to the formal academic preparation of nurses in the area of applications of computer technology and information science, nurses need to be educated in how to use the *specific* information technology germane to their practice environments.

One of the key requirements for successful utilization of any computerized health care system is to provide and enforce a thorough training program for personnel.[1] The results of a survey of staff development programs related to computer training in hospitals with computerized systems suggested that there is no single blueprint for training programs.[2]

---

[1] L. Guttman and S. Doyle, "Evolution of a Training Program for a Computerized Patient Data Management System," in *Proceedings of the Fifth Annual Symposium on Computer Applications in Medical Care*, ed. H. Heffernan (Los Angeles: Institute of Electrical and Electronics Engineers Computer Society, 1981), 772–779.

[2] S. Holloran, "Teaching a Computerized Patient Information System: State of the Art," in *Proceedings of the Sixth Annual Symposium for Computer Applications in Medical Care*, ed. B. Blum (Los Angeles: Institute of Electrical and Electronics Engineers Computer Society, 1982), 531–533.

Two themes were stressed in most of the programs surveyed, however: (1) involvement of system users in planning training sessions, and (2) open communication among all those affected by the system. In addition, the survey found that hospital-based education programs need to emphasize the rationale for instituting computerization and the benefits that the systems offer to nursing, the patient, and the hospital.

Research findings in the field of training users for computerized systems vary. Thoren reports that carefully planned, formal classroom educational programs are more likely to effect a smooth introduction to computer use.[3] Thies, in contrast, concludes that hospital personnel develop a greater understanding through experience derived from working demonstrations and self-instruction.[4] Guttman and Doyle report positive results from application of Thies's findings.[5]

The experience of educating over 2,000 nurses to use the computerized hospitalwide medical information system at the Clinical Center, the 550-bed research hospital of the National Institutes of Health, suggests that staff development programs in this area should combine the classroom and hands-on approaches of Thoren and Thies.[6] In addition, such a program should address all three learning domains: the cognitive, psychomotor, and affective. This paper describes the process of educating nurses in this clinical practice setting and shares strategies found to be successful in training.

CONTENT AND LEARNING STRATEGIES

The education program is designed to provide 26 hours of classroom instruction in two-hour daily sessions. Educational content is designed to prepare the user, through hands-on experiences, to gain access and use the computer technology in the clinical area. Instruction focuses on computer techniques for communicating with various hospital departments, the impact of the technology on traditional nursing activities, and issues of confidentiality.

Instruction methodologies include seminar sessions, self-paced written instruction modules, and reinforcement of learning by clinical unit preceptors. Each class session is "teacher facilitated" to add "touch" to the "high-tech" skills.

---

[3] J. T. Thoren, "Attitude Study, Training Helps Employees Adapt to Use of Computers," *Journal of the American Hospital Association* 43, no. 5 (1969):62.

[4] J. P. Thies, "Hospital Personnel and Computer Based Systems: A Study of Attitudes and Perceptions," *Hospital Administration* 1, no. 20 (1975): 24.

[5] Guttman and Doyle, "Evolution of a Training Program for a Computerized Patient Data Management System."

[6] C. Romano et al., "A Decade of Decisions: Four Perspectives of Computerization in Nursing Practice," *Computers in Nursing* 3 (March/April 1985): 64–76.

A special classroom designed to accommodate seven computer terminals and a printer is used for the instruction. Training software simulates a mock hospital, complete with nursing units, patients, doctors, and a patient information data base. Educational support is not restricted to the classroom, however. Follow-up support and resources for problem solving are available from the computer office staff as well as the nursing information system specialist and nurse educator.

PROGRAM PHASES

The psychomotor, cognitive, and affective learning domains are addressed in computer training at the Clinical Center through a four-phase educational approach. Phase 1 takes place during the first week of orientation and is coordinated by the nurse with accountability for computer systems and issues. Instruction focuses on an overview of the Clinical Center's computerized information system and on the "blueprint" for nursing process documentation.[7] Educational strategies during this phase are directed toward the affective learning domain, that is, dealing with changes in feeling, emotions, interests, attitudes, and degree of acceptance of computerization.[8] This introduction session was initiated at the request of learners, and follow-up evaluations confirm its value. The session provides the opportunity to defuse computer anxiety and to address preconceived misconceptions. It also prepares the learner for Phase 2.

Phase 2 is initiated during the second week of orientation and involves 16 hours of hands-on instruction. Computerized documentation and communication of interdependent nursing activities—those taken on the patient's behalf in response to the medical plan—are emphasized. Learning focuses on the fundamental skills required to access and navigate through the computerized nursing applications. The psychomotor skills of coordination and dexterity are also addressed through the exercises, which require the learner to interact with a computer terminal.

Phase 3 focuses on the cognitive skills of documenting the phases of the nursing process. A two-hour learning session is devoted to each of the following areas: (1) nursing assessment, (2) nursing diagnosis and patient care planning, (3) implementation and evaluation, and (4) discharge planning. Continuity of learning between the sessions is facilitated by the utilization of a case study. All sessions are conducted through hands-on computer exercises.

The final phase of the education process is a comprehensive evaluation

---

[7] C. Romano, "Documentation of Nursing Practice Using a Computerized Medical Information System," in *Proceedings of the Fifth Annual Symposium on Computer Applications in Medical Care*, 749–752.

[8] B. W. Narrow, "The Domains of Learning," *Patient Teaching in Nursing Practice: A Patient and Family-Centered Approach* (New York: John Wiley & Sons, 1979), 112–117.

of the effectiveness of the program. It includes input from both learners and instructors involved in each phase. Evaluation addresses learners' oral evaluations of the entire computer training experience, written self-assessments of each of the computer exercises in nursing process, and a nursing process audit of the learner's computerized documentation of patient care in the clinical setting.

SUMMARY

Complex and extensive computerized clinical nursing applications clearly require preparation of the users. What is less obvious, however, is that user training involves instruction in two areas. Both the *how* of manipulating and handling the computer hardware and software and the *who*, *when*, *where*, and *why* of specific applications must be addressed. The nurse educator should recognize, however, that the time dedicated to computer instruction in nursing orientation and staff development programs need not necessarily be added on to hours already devoted to current orientation programs. Traditional educational sessions directed toward introducing employees to hospital policies and information-handling procedures may not be necessary if this material is incorporated into the computer classes.

Educational programs need to be developed and delivered efficiently and effectively. The strategies addressed in this paper for implementing computer technology in nursing have proved to be successful. The role of nursing education in smoothing the transition to the skillful use of computerization in health care is critical.

CURRENT RESEARCH ON COMPUTER USE IN NURSING

GARY D. HALES, PhD
Editor in Chief, *Computers in Nursing*
Software Editor, J. B. Lippincott Company
Houston, Texas

One of the more frustrating aspects of dealing with computers in education or in applied settings is that one must answer the critics who state, sometimes quite eloquently, that computers are not really that useful. Pointing out the learning curve for some software, the doubters make a good point for maintaining traditional methods. Indeed, for the advocate of computer use in nursing, one of the greatest hurdles to overcome is the enthusiasm expressed by others. There are still those who, subsequent to their first exposure to the computer and computer-assisted instruction (CAI), for example, feel that it is a panacea—that the computer, with accompanying software, is likely to correct many of the problems of poorly designed curriculum that can plague a program. This naive view is rapidly diminishing as evidence mounts that computerizing a curriculum results in no more change than the addition of new tools. Old mistakes in curriculum design, planning, and topic selection may be highlighted by the changeover process, but will not be automatically corrected.

This paper will describe some studies and examine some trends in computer use in nursing education and practice. My purpose is not to provide an exhaustive review of this literature, but rather to pique the reader's interest and provide a starting point for the reader's own review of the literature.

CURRENT TRENDS IN THE LITERATURE

Examination of the writings from the published proceedings of recent conferences, from published and submitted journal articles, and from compilations of materials, such as the annotated bibliography by Pocklington and Guttman, produces four basic categories of articles.[1] At one end of the continuum are the "hard research" articles and, at the other end, those that may be classified as philosophical/anecdotal in nature. This review will start at the latter end of the spectrum.

Philosophical/Anecdotal Articles

One of the problems that has concerned nursing in its use of computers evolves from the training of the nurses who are reporting on computer use. Until recently, the training that graduate nursing students received in research methodology was, in most cases, insufficient to prepare them to design and conduct research and use appropriate statistical techniques to analyze the data. Instead, students and faculty members were forced to rely on the expertise and biases of social scientists for these tasks. Due at least in part to these deficiencies, a great deal of the literature involving computer use in nursing falls into the category of interesting personal position papers that cannot be generalized to any other situation.

In this category are papers with titles like "Computers: What Do They Mean to Nursing?" that, while presenting some very good ideas, rely for their facts on the opinions of one or two or more people who have "discovered" computers and wish to state their opinion in a wider forum than the faculty lounge. There is a definite place for such publications, of course, since combining the newest technology with an established discipline requires not only the act of doing so, but also the planning necessary to make the transition logical if not smooth. Examples of articles falling in this category are McHugh and Shultz's paper on applications of computer technology in hospital nursing departments; Saba's description of computer use in nursing education, administration, research, and practice; and Jacobsen and Fennell's article on using the systems life cycle concept to manage computer implementation.[2] In fact, when Pock-

---

[1] D. B. Pocklington and L. Guttman, *Nursing Reference for Computer Literature* (Philadelphia: J. B. Lippincott Co., 1984).

[2] M. McHugh and S. Schultz, "Computer Technology in Hospital Nursing Departments: Future Applications and Implications," in *Proceedings of the Sixth Annual Symnposium on Computer Applications in Medical Care*, ed. B. Blum (Los Angeles: Institute of Electrical and Electronics Engineers Computer Society, 1982), 557–561; and V. K. Saba, "Computer Applications in Nursing," and T. J. Jacobsen and S. E. Fennell, "Systems Life Cycle: Strategy for Managing the Impact of Information Systems on Nursing," 469–471, both in *Proceedings of the Seventh Annual Symposium on Computer Applications in Medical Care*, ed. R. E. Dayhoff (Los Angeles: Institute of Electrical and Electronics Engineers Computer Society, 1983).

lington and Guttman classifed articles on computer use in nursing, they indicated that the majority of the articles examined fell into their "general" category, which, from a cursory examination of the abstracts, reflects what I am calling philosophical/anecdotal material. The proceedings from the past three Symposia on Computer Applications in Medical Care (SCAMC) also show a preponderance of philosophical/anecdotal articles on use and articles on applications of computers.

Applications

The articles on applications of computers are one step up and one step over from the purely philosophical/anecdotal papers. Although such articles often present a personal position about the need for, abuse of, and use of computers, at least in this case the use of particular systems are described, compared, or otherwise exemplified. This has a potentially positive outcome, since the reader is cautioned against reinventing the wheel. Although the information presented is usually based on a single case study, the reader is at least given the benefit of someone's practical experience. Some examples of articles of this type include Newbern's description of a continuing education course; Hardin and Skiba's article on tailoring educational modes to best address specific computer literacy needs by nurses; Roehrl, Nickel, and Lake's paper on using patient classification data collection forms to estimate staffing needs; Weaver and Johnson's discussion of how nurses can be active and primary participants in selecting vendors of hospital information systems; Skiba and Hardin on using microcomputers in computer workshops; Holzemer et al.'s report of the development of a microcomputer facility for nursing research; Redland and Kilmon on developing interactive video; and Light's description of the development of a hospital information system.[3] The problem remains, however, that one cannot generalize these experiences outside of the restricted conditions prevailing in the environs in which the activity took place.

---

[3] V. B. Newbern, "Introducing Computer Content in Nursing Education: One Experience," 516–519, R. C. Hardin and D. J. Skiba, "A Comparative Analysis of Computer Literacy Education for Nurses, 524–530, and P. K. Roehrl, L. L. Nickel, and W. H. Lake, "Nurse Staffing through Patient Classification," 551–556, all in *Proceedings of the Sixth Annual Symposium on Computer Applications in Medical Care*; C. G. Weaver and J. E. Johnson, "Nursing Participation in Computer Vendor Selection," *Computers in Nursing* 2 (January/February 1984): 31–34; D. J. Skiba and R. C. Hardin, "Development and Implementation of a Micro-based Computer Workshop Series for Nurses," 480–483; and W. L. Holzemer, M. J. Slichter, R. E. Slaughter, and N. A. Stotts, "Development of the University of California, San Francisco, Microcomputer Facility for Nursing Research and Development, 484–486, both in *Proceedings of the Seventh Annual Symposium on Computer Applications in Medical Care*; A. R. Redland and C. Kilmon, "Interactive Video: Rationale and Practicalities of One Experience," in *Proceedings of the First Annual Conference on Computer-Assisted Interactive Video Instruction* (Sacramento: Division of Nursing, California State University, Sacramento, 1985); and N. Light, "Developing a Hospital Information System Nursing Database," in *Proceedings of the Second National Conference on Computer Technology and Nursing*, ed. R. Carlson (Washington, D.C.: Clinical Center Office of Clinical Reports and Inquiries, National Institutes of Health, 1982), 663–667.

Research

The least represented area of writing in computers in nursing is research—studies using experimental or quasi-experimental designs to provide the reader not only with information but also with the methods to attempt to replicate the original findings or at least with some confidence that the findings may be generalized beyond a very specific situation. Again, the category with the fewest articles in Pocklington and Guttman's bibliography is that of research. Examination of, among other sources, the most recent SCAMC proceedings and articles submitted to *Computers in Nursing* yields the following topics for research articles:

- Use of the technology in dedicated devices for data collection: Abbey and Close describe use of telemonitoring and computer controlled data monitoring; and Thompson discusses using a pocket programmable computer to calculate routine patient assessment parameters.[4]

- Survey research regarding computer use on clinical units: Marticelli and Fisher discuss preferred data input methods; and Milholland and Brady report on user satisfaction with a computerized interactive critical care data base.[5]

- Comparison of traditional versus computer aided methods of patient monitoring: discussed by Milholland and Ward.[6]

- Development of systems to improve nursing care decision making, reported by Ozbolt.[7]

- Effectiveness of CAI: Larson presents the results of a study of teaching effectiveness and efficiency with CAI; and Murphy discusses various factors influencing the effectiveness of CAI.[8]

---

[4] J. C. Abbey and L. Close, "Impact of Technological Research on Nursing Practice," in *Proceedings of the Sixth Annual Symposium on Computer Applications in Medical Care*, 593–596; and D. A. Thompson, "Monitoring Total Parenteral Nutrition with the Pocket Computer," *Computers in Nursing* 2 (September/October): 183–188.

[5] B. Marticelli and S. G. Fisher, "A Study of the Utilization of the Automated Patient Reassessment Component of a Medical Information System," in *Proceedings of the Sixth Annual Symposium on Computer Applications in Medical Care*, 597–607; and K. Milholland and L. Brady, "Clinical Staff Satisfaction with a Computerized Critical Care Database System," in *Seventh Annual Symposium on Computer Applications in Medical Care*, 516–518.

[6] K. Milholland and J. M. Ward, "A Comparison of Computer Recorded and Manually Recorded Heart Rates and Systolic Blood Pressure," in *Proceedings of the Sixth Annual Symposium on Computer Applications in Medical Care*, 608–611.

[7] J. G. Ozbolt, "A Prototype Information System to Aid Nursing Decisions," in *Proceedings of the Sixth Annual Symposium on Computer Applications in Medical Care*, 653–657.

[8] D. E. Larson, "Microcomputer Tutorial-Simulations to Teach Basic Nursing Skills," in *Proceedings of the Sixth Annual Symposium on Computer Applications in Medical Care*, 663–667; and M. A. Murphy, "Computer-Based Education in Nursing; Factors Affecting its Utilization," *Computers in Nursing* 2 (November-December 1984): 218–223.

- Using and evaluating new technologies in nursing: Sparks, Mirr and Golembrewski report on an interactive video.[9]

- Studies regarding nurse acceptance of computers: by nurse educators (Ronald); by hospital nurses (Chang, Jordan-Marsh, and Chang, and Jordan-Marsh and Chang); by learners (Ball, Snelbecker, and Schechter); and by students and faculty (Stronge and Brodt). Pillar reports on the measurement of technology anxiety.[10]

- Survey research on computer use in diverse areas of nursing: Johnson did a survey of administrative use (in the dean's office); and Thomas surveyed computer use in nursing education.[11]

- Use of new technologies in nursing: Edwards and Hannah examine the use of interactive video in cardiopulmonary resuscitation; Rickelman et al. discuss interactive video and reduction of anxiety; Meehan-Longcrier studied interactive video in nursing education; Allen, Devney, and Sharpe report on error detection taught through computer-assisted interactive video instruction (CAIVI); and Fishman presents the use of CAIVI to teach cancer chemotherapy to nurses.[12]

- Instrument development: Skaggs and Kilmon report on the formative evaluation of interactive video; and Wallace, Slichter, and Bolwell describe the development of an assessment device for CAI.[13]

---

[9] R. K. Sparks, M. Mirr, and I. Golembiewski, "Nursing Care of the Acute Trauma Patient: An Interactive Video Program," in *Proceedings of the First Annual Conference on Computer-Assisted Interactive Video Instruction.*

[10] J. Ronald, "Learning Needs and Attitudes of Nurse Education with Respect to Computers," 523–527, and B. L. Chang, M. Jordan-Marsh, and A. F. Chang, "Nursing Expectations of Computers in the Hospital," 519–522, both in *Proceedings of the Seventh Annual Symposium on Computer Applications in Medical Care*; M. Jordan-Marsh and B. L. Chang, "Assessing Readiness for Interaction with Computers in Medical Centers," *Computers in Nursing* (in press); M. J. Ball, G. E. Snelbecker, and S. L. Schechter, "Nurses' Perceptions Concerning Computer Use Before and After a Computer Literacy Lecture," *Computers in Nursing* 3 (January/February 1985): 23–32; J. H. Stronge and A. Brodt, "Assessment of Nurses' Attitudes Toward Computerization," *Computers in Nursing* (in press); and B. Pillar, "The Measurement of Technology Anxiety," unpublished ms. (1985).

[11] B. M. Johnson, "Microcomputers in the Nursing Dean's Office," in *Proceedings of the Seventh Annual Symposium on Computer Applications in Medical Care*, 528; and B. S. Thomas, "A Survey Study of Computers in Nursing Education," *Computers in Nursing* (in press).

[12] M. J. A. Edwards and K. Hannah, "An Examination of the Use of Interactive Videodisc Cardiopulmonary Resuscitation Instruction for the Lay Community," B. L. Rickelman et al., "Impact of a Computer Video Interactive System (CVIS) Instructional Program Regarding Therapeutic Communication on Student Anxiety and Learning," N. Meehan-Longcrier, "A Study of the Effectiveness of Interactive Video in Nursing Education," and B. S. Allen, A. M. Devney, and D. M. Sharpe, "The Effect of Error Detection Practice on Performance of a Simple Medical Procedure," all in *Proceedings of the First Annual Conference on Computer-Assisted Interactive Video Instruction*; and D. Fishman, "Development and Evaluation of a Computer Assisted Video Module for Teaching Cancer Chemotherapy to Nurses," *Computers in Nursing* 2 (January/February 1984): 16–23.

[13] B. J. Skaggs and C. A. Kilmon, "Formative Evaluation of Computer Interactive Video Program: User Component," in *Proceedings of the First Annual Conference on Computer-Assisted Interactive Video Instruction*; and D. Wallace, M. Slichter, and C. Bolwell, "Evaluation Criteria for CAI Courseware: A Psychometric Approach," unpublished ms. (1985).

- Evaluation of systems: discussed by Farlee.[14]

The research studies that are now beginning to appear in the area of computer use in nursing suggest some major trends. First, studies are still being done to determine if CAI in general can be beneficial. It would seem to be much more productive for nurse educators to devote their research time to investigating specific computer uses in clinical nursing and nursing education. It would be useful, for example, to study the inservice or continuing education impact of computers for training and to examine if CAI is more productive in cognitive, affective, or psychomotor areas.

Another trend in the literature is the development of instrumentation of two specific kinds. The first is the development of tools to assess the effectiveness of software, whether educational or applications oriented. It could be said that this is really the province of the educational psychologist or educational researcher. To a certain extent, all well-written software shares certain characteristics; to this degree, the nurse researcher can borrow from other disciplines. When the content is very specific to nursing, however, the nurse researcher should inject those items that uniquely describe nursing situations and considerations.

The second type of instrumentation is the attitude survey. In time it will become trivial, at best, to measure the attitudes of nurses toward using computers in different settings since they will be knowledgeable about computer systems to begin with—just as they are knowledgeable about microwave ovens and toasters now. At this point, however, it is important to be concerned with the feelings of users and potential users in order to expedite the implementation of computers.

It also becomes very important to begin to bring research methodology to bear on the evaluation of the implementation of nursing and hospital systems and of peripheral software. Rather than simply report that an *XYZ* system was implemented in such-and-such a way, it is incumbent on the nurse administrator to undertake or to assign someone to utilize at least a quasi-experimental design, to survey users before and after implementation, or to assess the meeting of objectives (before and after) to determine the effectiveness of a particular system. This research should occur simultaneously with the formative and summative evaluation of the computer implementation. It is economically valuable in that it provides justification for further expansion or expenditures in other more profitable areas. In addition, by sharing such information, colleagues can avoid making the same mistakes and can beneift from each other's experience.

The impact of brand new technologies—interactive video, telecom-

---

[14] C. Farlee, "Systems Evaluation: Problems and Challenges," in *Proceedings of the First National Conference on Computer Technology and Nursing*, ed. R. Carlson (Washington, D.C.: Clinical Center Office of Clinical Reports and Inquiries, National Institutes of Health, 1981), 34–41.

munications, portability of systems and software, and expert systems—should be studied to determine their current, short-term, and long-term effects on nursing and nursing practice. Some research has been done in these areas, either by intent or default. In some cases, the nurse researcher is reporting on work done to examine the effects of new technology that has been inserted into his or her work environment and now must be assessed. Ideally, the nurse researcher would have the opportunity to do some kind of pilot study prior to implementation in order to determine before-and-after differences or at least establish some sort of baseline data from which to determine effectiveness.

RESEARCH METHODOLOGIES

The types of methodologies used to examine the use of computers in nursing typically fall into the following categories: small case study, attitude measurement, development or use of assessment devices, experimental and quasi-experimental designs, survey research, and evaluation studies. The small case studies, with the exception noted later, supply additional fuel to anecdotal reporting of the wonders or disasters of computerization but provide very little hard evidence for advantages or disadvantages.

Of greater import are studies utilizing survey methods to (1) determine acceptance of computers in various areas of nursing, and (2) determine use of computers in various areas of nursing. The predisposition of the individuals who are being ushered into the computer age, the amount and type of training they receive, and the support system established for them contribute directly to the immediate or long-term success of computer implementation. By determining the point at which the potential users start, one may map out a strategy for addressing real and imagined fears. Of equal importance are surveys that are designed to assess implementation of certain systems—that is, the use of computers in a large area of nursing, for example, the number of installed computers being used for CAI in baccalaureate schools.

Of most interest and of greatest use are studies that use evaluation methodology or classical experimental design to generate results that may be generalized with confidence and relied on as a basis for further study. These types of studies are, unfortunately, also in shortest supply.

Although I would not consider it a valid research methodology, an important aspect of assessing the effectiveness of computers in nursing is the report made by users regarding implementation of a system. In this case, the users, while not employing scientific methods, take copious notes on the problems and solutions, the highs and lows, and the ins and outs of moving a system from the conceptualization to the implementation. Optimally, formative and summative evaluation data would be collected on such implementation, but often the reporting is quite anecdotal. Even so, since the information is practical and specific to particular computer and software configurations, it can be very valuable.

Whatever methodology is used, it is becoming increasingly important for nurse researchers to examine the impact of computer use in nursing from their unique perspective as triple professionals—as trained nurses, researchers, and computer users.

NEED FOR RESEARCH ON COMPUTER USE

Without referring to findings based on research, the claims and counter-claims for the use of computers in nursing education, practice, research, and administration have equal weight. Justification for actions becomes a matter of who can speak the loudest and longest rather than who has the best rationales and support. In addition, current research inevitably inspires further research and increases the chances for locating funding sources. Examining in minute detail the use of computers suggests new uses of computers. It is only in this way that one can validate or invalidate the claims and counterclaims made for computer use in nursing.

COMPUTER-ASSISTED DECISION MAKING IN THE NURSING PROCESS

WILLIAM L. HOLZEMER, PhD
Associate Professor, School of Nursing
University of California, San Francisco

Educators are intrigued with the complexity of the process of decision making in the clinical setting. Researchers have contributed to an extensive literature on clinical problem solving in nursing.[1] Reflecting recognition that decision making is a core phenomenon in nursing, their work has focused on theory development, measurement strategies, techniques for improving decision making, and alternative methodologies for examining this phenomenon.

Research on clinical decision making is based on conceptualizations of the nursing process, "the application of scientific problem solving to nursing care."[2] Today, the concept of nursing diagnosis has been incorporated into the nursing process as a mechanism to describe clients' actual or potential health problems. Nursing process and diagnosis both imply clinical decision making.

---

[1] See, for example, J. Bailey, F. J. McDonald, and K. E. Claus, *An Experiment in Nursing Curriculums at a University* (Belmont, Calif.: Wadsworth Publishing, 1971); M. R. Grier, "Decision-Making about Patient Care," *Nursing Research* 25 (1976): 105–110; C. A. Tanner, "Research on Clinical Judgment," in *Review of Research in Nursing Education*, ed. W. L. Holzemer, Vol. 1 (Thorofare, N.J.: C. B. Slack, 1983), 2–32; and P. Benner, *From Novice to Expert: Excellence and Power in Clinical Nursing Practice* (Menlo Park, Calif.: Addison-Wesley, 1984).

[2] A. Marriner, *The Nursing Process: A Scientific Approach to Nursing Care* (St. Louis, Mo.: C. V. Mosby, 1983), 1.

Nursing is now witnessing the development of computer systems to aid decision making in the clinical arena. This paper presents an overview of computer-assisted decision making (CADM) within the framework of clinical problem-solving and nursing diagnosis.

NURSING PROCESS/NURSING DIAGNOSIS

The nursing process is the cornerstone of professional nursing practice. Used universally in nursing education to help students understand and organize the delivery of nursing care, the nursing process is used less formally by nurses in practice. According to Yura and Walsh, the

> nursing process is an orderly, systematic manner of determining the client's problems, making plans to solve them, initiating the plan or assigning others to implement it, and evaluating the extent to which the plan was effective in resolving the problems identified.[3]

Tanner describes the cognitive activity involved in the nursing process as "a linear sequence of thought processes which includes the steps of assessment, planning, intervention, and evaluation."[4] The *Social Policy Statement* of the American Nurses' Association presents the nursing process as a five-part process including data collection, diagnosis, planning, treatment, and evaluation.[5]

The nursing process can be conceptualized for both educational and practice settings. Specifically, it provides a step-by-step sequence of events particularly helpful to the nursing student or new graduate in organizing and structuring the assessment, planning, treatment, and evaluation activities of nursing care. The nursing process also has applicability for the experienced nurse in the sense that it represents a strategy for problem solving that is generalizable across states of health and illness, clients, and settings.

Because of the need to establish a common framework for the identification of client problems addressed in nursing, nurses began the development of nursing diagnosis. Gordon defines nursing diagnoses as "actual or potential health problems which nurses by virtue of their education and experience are capable and licensed to treat."[6] The development of this common nomenclature allows clinicians in diverse settings to label

---

[3] H. Yura and M. B. Walsh, *The Nursing Process: Assessing, Planning, Implementing, Evaluating*, 3d ed. (New York: Appleton-Century-Crofts, 1978), p. 20.

[4] Tanner, "Research on Clinical Judgment," 2.

[5] *Nursing: A Social Policy Statement* (Kansas City, Mo.: American Nurses' Association, 1980), 14–15.

[6] M. Gordon, *Nursing Diagnosis: Process and Application* (New York: McGraw-Hill Book Co., 1982), 2.

commonly occurring collections of clinical signs and symptoms of interest to nursing in a formal, organized fashion. Although under continual development, the current listing of 50 nursing diagnoses provides a structure that can be utilized by a computer-assisted decision-making system to organize information for nursing administration, practice, and research.[7] Nursing diagnosis was not originally specified as a component of the nursing process. Today, however, the assessment step of the nursing process is acknowledged to include both data collection and diagnosis, followed by the steps of planning, treatment, and evaluation.

Within the steps of the nursing process, the number of potential decision points is staggering. The nurse is continually making decisions based on input and feedback from the client, the context, and other factors. Given the complexity of the decision-making process, can computer systems be used to improve the quality and accuracy of decision making within nursing? How can a computer help one to be a better nurse? A description of computer-assisted decision-making systems will provide a framework for exploring the potential use of such computer systems in clinical decision making in nursing.

COMPUTERS: WHAT CAN THEY DO?

When several nursing colleagues were informally surveyed regarding their impressions of what computers could do, they responded with the observation that computers had good memories and could accurately recall facts. One saw the computer as an encyclopedia that stored information of interest to her. Another spoke of how computers could "crunch" numbers for report writing and statistical analyses. A third mentioned that computers were great at keeping lists of things. Still another mentioned that computers were excellent for repetitive tasks such as sending personalized form letters or typing multiple copies of original-looking manuscripts.

To this list of computer skills—keeping lists, "crunching" numbers, excellent memory, and ease of accomplishing repetitive tasks—a few additional characteristics need to be added. These include vastly increasing speeds for accomplishing operations; significantly reduced costs for providing services; sophisticated graphics; voice recognition and voice synthesizing; networking, or computers talking with each other; real-time monitoring of physiological phenomena such as blood gases and vital signs; robotics, or the machine-human interfaces; optical scanning of the

---

[7] *Ibid.*

printed word; interactive video; and the focus of this paper, computer-assisted decision making (CADM).

Considering that microprocessors (computer chips) are now found not only in computers but also in watches, automobiles, hearing aids, and experimentally in prosthetic devices, one might well question just what a computer is. In light of the many uses of microprocessors, it is necessary to expand the concept of the computer. Although more and more products today are enhanced with microprocessors, however, the computer has traditionally been viewed as a data-processing device. For purposes of this paper, computer-assisted decision making will be considered within the traditional framework of the computer as "a data processing device that can perform substantial computation, including numerous arithemetic or logic operations without intervention by a human operator during the processing."[8] Nevertheless, the expert systems and artificial intelligence systems of CADM reflect a less traditional application of the computer as a data-processing device.

The business world uses the term *decision support systems* (DSS) to refer to the capacity computers have to help with decisions. In the health field, the term *computer-assisted decision making* or CADM is popular. CADM systems will be classified here as support systems, expert systems, and artificial intelligence systems, based on the degree to which they actually represent qualities of human decision-making processes.

SUPPORT SYSTEMS

Support systems utilize the capacities of the computer in sophisticated, yet understandable ways. Support systems are used for managing, modeling, monitoring, communicating, and analyzing data. A few examples are presented here to show systems in current use and applications predicted for the near future.

Managing Systems

A managing system is commonly a data-base application, such as an acuity care system that relates patients' levels of illness to staffing requirements. A common microcomputer software for this type of system is DBASE III. Based on the acuity level of patients on a unit, a computer-based support system can evaluate staffing requirements quickly and consistently and make recommendations to increase or decrease the level of nurse staffing. Managing systems of the future will include tele-

---

[8] J. O'Brien, *Computers in Business Management* (Homewood, Ill.: Richard D. Irwin, 1982), 655.

communication devices to allow easy communication among diverse data bases.

Modeling Systems

Another type of support system is the modeling system—a system that can predict outcomes based on hypothetical data. One application is for fiscal purposes, such as using personnel records that include hours worked along with salary and benefits costs to predict costs of changing staffing patterns. Lotus 1-2-3 is a common microcomputer software package for this function. Different financial models for costing out nursing services can be made for the nurse executive based on different staffing requirements, given varying salary and benefit levels. In the practice arena, modeling systems or "what-if" simulators will eventually allow the clinician to simulate different nursing interventions and then to assess the alternative client outcomes.

Monitoring Systems

The use of monitoring systems for decision making in intensive care and critical care units is quite common today. These systems have the ability to collect data in real time—that is, while phenomena such as blood pressure, pulse, and temperature are actually occurring—and follow "alarm rules" to notify nurses of the patient's condition. Alarm rules are mechanisms to assist decision making, for example, setting an acceptable range for the pulse so that if the patient's pulse moves above or below that value, an alarm is triggered. These systems are also used to monitor episodes of sleep apnea. In the future, home monitoring systems will be developed to assist the visiting nurse in assessment, management, communication, and follow-up with a client in his or her home.

Communicating Systems

Communicating systems allow the user to access data available in diverse settings by linking several data bases together. A hospital pharmacy system can be linked through a communication system to a national drug information system, allowing a staff nurse to search for interactions and side effects of a medication about to be administered. Communication systems allow the utilization of relational data bases—that is, having the ability to combine information from unrelated data bases—to improve decision making. The future will bring these systems into the day-to-day practice of all health care providers at much lower costs.

Analyzing Systems

Analyzing systems are commonly statistical packages such as the Statistical Package for the Social Sciences (SPSS), which are now available for the microcomputer. These systems allow the researcher to present data in a parsimonious fashion, using such statistics as means and standard deviations as descriptors of a sample. Future market policies will lower the cost for these software packages and improve both their accuracy and ease of use.

Support systems, the first category of computer-assisted decision making, include functions such as managing, modeling, monitoring, communicating, and analyzing. These support systems are available now for enhancing decision making for nurse clinicians, educators, administrators, and researchers. The nursing profession is moving rapidly to incorporate the advantages of these computer-assisted decision-making systems into every aspect of nursing.

EXPERT SYSTEMS

An expert system may be defined as "a computer program that performs a specialized, usually difficult professional task at the level of (or sometimes beyond the level of) a human expert."[9] Kunz et al. outline five types of CADM expert systems that have current applications primarily for medical decision making.[10] Four of these types of systems are included in this section, and the fifth, artificial intelligence, is here treated as a distinct category and is discussed separately.

The first type of expert system uses clinical algorithms such as flowcharts or protocols. These systems use "if-then" conditions to provide guidelines for practice. For example, Goldman et al. report a data bank for managing patients who complain of common chest pain.[11] Computer algorithms have been used with physician assistants.[12] Protocols based on similar "if-then" reasoning, although not computerized, are common in settings where nurse practitioners handle problems with indirect medical supervision. In the future, algorithms to computerize nursing protocols will be developed.

The second type of expert system is statistical analysis of patient data. These systems have been developed with the goal of medical diagnosis.

---

[9] E. A. Feigenbaum and P. McCorduck, *The Fifth Generation: Artificial Intelligence and Japan's Computer Challenge to the World* (Reading, Mass.: Addison-Wesley, 1984), p. 312.

[10] J. C. Kunz et al., "Computer-Assisted Decision-Making in Medicine," *Journal of Medicine and Philosophy* 9 (1984): 135–160.

[11] L. Goldman et al., "A Computer-Derived Protocol to Aid in the Diagnosis of Emergency Room Patients with Acute Chest Pain," *New England Journal of Medicine* 307 (1982): 588–596.

[12] S. R. Cannon and R. M. Gardner, "Experience with a Computerized Interactive Protocol System Using HELP," *Computers & Biomedical Research* 13 (1980): 399–409.

Given certain signs and symptoms, the probability of having a particular disease can be quickly calculated and presented with a certain confidence interval. For example, deDombal et al. report that a Bayesian statistical computer program outperformed physicians in diagnosing the causes of abdominal pain.[13] This type of expert system can be particularly helpful as a learning tool for new health care professionals or isolated professionals presented with a rare combination of signs and symptoms. As empirical research becomes available to document that a cluster of patients' signs and symptoms are consistently associated with certain nursing diagnoses, similar probability or statistical analysis systems will be developed to predict nursing diagnoses. Corresponding nursing care plans will also be available, given the nursing diagnosis.

A third type of expert system uses mathematical models to represent physical processes. Such systems are found today in fields such as pharmacy and toxicology. Decisions about the feasibility of combining various chemical elements can be determined based on these computer-assisted graphic models. When Gorry, Silverman, and Pauker compared the performance of clinicians and a computer program in digitalis therapy, in all cases where digitalis toxicity developed, the computer program would have recommended a lower dosage.[14]

The fourth model is a refinement of the second and third systems and is referred to as Bayes theory decision analysis. Signs and symptoms are assigned probabilities of independent and dependent occurrences. Given an observation of a specific combination of signs and symptoms, certain diagnoses can be determined with specific probability confidences.

These four models of expert systems are not well represented in nursing. Several such systems have been developed in medicine, but few, if any, are actually used outside the research and development environment.[15] These CADM systems tend to consist of rule-based or "if-then" statements of facts and relationships. The systems operate not as a human expert is hypothesized to operate, but rather as a data-processing device, a computer. In contrast, the human expert is not someone who just follows rules. He or she has the experience that enables recognition of the unusual. How people think and how they perform is not adequately represented in these rule-based models of expert systems. Artificial intelligence systems—what Kunz et al. referred to as the fifth type of expert system—attempt to capture the unique dimensions of symbolic reasoning and are sometimes referred to as the fifth generation of computers.

---

[13] F. T. deDombal et al., "Human and Computer-Aided Diagnosis of Abdominal Pain: Further Report with Emphasis on Performance of Clinicians," *British Medical Journal* 1 (1974): 376–380.

[14] G. A. Gorry, H. Silverman, and S. G. Pauker, "Capturing Clinical Expertise: A Computer Program that Considers Clinical Responses to Digitalis," *American Journal of Medicine* 64 (1978): 452–460.

[15] W. J. Clancey and E. H. Shortliffe, *Readings in Artificial Intelligence* (Reading, Mass.: Addison-Wesley Publishing Co., 1984).

ARTIFICIAL INTELLIGENCE

Artificial intelligence (AI) systems are open decision-support systems that have the capacity to change and evolve. They have a memory of their own behavior, representation of their procedures for interacting with the external world, and an ability to tolerate inconsistencies in their knowledge structure.[16] Scientists suggest that useful AI systems will be able to explain and justify what they do, communicate well with both people and other expert systems, restructure and reorganize knowledge, break rules, determine relevance of information to the question at hand, and degrade (shut down) gracefully. MYCIN was one of the first systems to approach the characteristics of an AI system.[17] The goal of MYCIN is to make diagnoses and recommend therapy for patients suffering from infectious diseases. Another AI system in medicine is INTERNIST-1, which assists with diagnosis and ordering of tests for all diseases in internal medicine.[18]

Feldman has written that "The field of AI is nowhere near possessing the ability to simulate the natural intelligence of a small child or even a simple animal."[19] For example, to simulate 10 milliseconds of the complete processing accomplished by even a single nerve cell from the retina would require the solution of about 500 simultaneous nonlinear differential equations 100 times and would take at least several minutes of process time on the Cray computer, the most powerful supercomputer available today. Moreover, there are 10 million or so such cells in the retina, and this translates into 100 person-years of supercomputer processing time to simulate what takes place in one individual's eye many times every second.[20]

The hypothetical AI system consists of three parts. First, there is a *knowledge base* composed of facts and rules about a phenomenon, such as patient signs and symptoms and diagnoses. This knowledge base is similar to that used in other expert systems. Second, an *inference engine* uses the reasoning process of a logical chaining mechanism to search, update, relate, revise, and explore the knowledge base. Third, these two components are addressed with a friendly *user interface* that understands the English language.

The schematic diagram presented in Figure 1 represents the hypothesized relationships among nursing process, nursing diagnosis, and the

---

[16] R. H. Michaelsen, D. Michie, and A. Boulanger, "The Technology of Expert Systems," *Byte* 10 (April 1985): 304.

[17] E. H. Shortliffe, *Computer-Based Medical Consultation: MYCIN* (New York: Elsevier/North Holland, 1976).

[18] R. A. Miller, H. E. Pople, and J. D. Myers, "INTERNIST-1, An Experimental Computer-Based Diagnostic Consultant for General Internal Medicine," *New England Journal of Medicine* 307 (1982): 468–476.

[19] J. A. Feldman, "Artificial Intelligence: Connections," *Byte* 10, no. 4 (1985): 277.

[20] J. K. Stevens, "Artificial Intelligence: Reverse Engineering the Brain," *Byte* 10, no. 4 (1985), 287–299.

Figure 1. Relationship among Nursing Process, Nursing Diagnosis, and Artificial Intelligence Systems

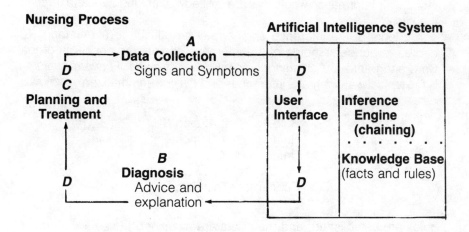

Nursing Process

A = Data collection (Signs and symptoms)
B = Diagnosis (ineffective individual coping leads to homebound status)
C = Planning and treatment (nursing home care services)
D = Evaluation (feedback loops)

Adapted from B.G. Buchanan and E. H. Shortliffe, *Rule-Based Expert Systems: The MYCIN Experiments of the Stanford Heuristic Programming Project* (Reading, Mass: Addison-Wesley Publishing Co., 1984), 4.

three parts of the AI system. Signs and symptoms for the data collection step are entered into the system either by the user interface or perhaps through a direct monitoring system. Based on the results of the inference engine's interaction with the knowledge base, a diagnosis, along with explanations appropriate for the observed signs and symptoms, would result. This information would then be utilized in planning care and treating the client.

The logic of the inference engine may be difficult to understand. To capture an understanding of the inference engine, the concepts of forward and backward chaining logic must be reviewed. *Forward chaining* is the typical way we make inferences and may be summarized as follows:

> Rule 1:   If A, then B
> Rule 2:   If B, then C
> Data: A
> _____
> Conclusion: Therefore C

Rules are established, and then data are examined to see if they meet the requirements of the rules. For example, Rule 1 might state that if an individual has certain signs and symptoms (A in Figure 1), then one can conclude that the individual has ineffective coping and may be classified as meeting federal regulations for homebound status (B). Rule 2 might suggest that if a client has homebound status (B), then certain nursing home care services (C) are required. If the data or signs and symptoms are present, the conclusion is drawn that nursing home services are required. Forward chaining logic is represented in the linear logic of the nursing process.

AI systems tend to function through *backward chaining* logic, which is summarized as follows:

> Goal: Find out about C
> Rule 1:   If B, then C
> Rule 2:   If A, then B
> _____
> Implicit Rule: Therefore if A, then C
> Question: Is A true? (Data)

First, a goal is set, which in this example is to find out whether home care services (C) are required. The two rules are the same. There is an implicit rule that states that if there is a given set of signs and symptoms, then the diagnosis of homebound status is justified. The AI system seeks to find out if A is true—that is, whether the signs and symptoms exist.[21] Therefore, the user interface would seek evidence to validate the existence and accuracy of the signs and symptoms.

The two types of chaining logic are important because they represent two different conceptual views of the world in problem solving. Forward chaining attempts to verify the conclusion, whereas backward chaining attempts to verify if the data (signs and symptoms) are true. Backward chaining assumes that there is a knowledge base from which to operate. It will be impossible for nursing to develop AI systems based on backward chaining until sufficient knowledge exists about the relationships among signs and symptoms, diagnoses, interventions, and evaluations.

AI AND NURSING

Two projects in nursing currently purport to be AI systems. The oldest is the COMMES (Creighton On-line Multiple Modular Expert System) project at Creighton University.[22] This system may best be conceptualized as a knowledge data base about the interrelationships among signs and symptoms of human conditions. It is not a nursing system per se, but rather an entire health care system based on client signs and symptoms. Its most apparent application is as an extensive information resource to consult with regarding a particular patient's signs and symptoms. Nursing diagnoses have been built into the system as well as optimal care plans, nursing interventions, and evaluation guidelines. The degree to which the system truly reflects the characteristics outlined here for an AI system as opposed to an expert system is unclear.

A second group has been working at the University of Michigan, headed by nurse researcher Dr. Judy Ozbolt.[23] Their current project is the development of an AI system for nursing practice in the area of elimination needs of the elderly person. They are attempting to combine a heuristic approach with a probabilistic expert system approach. It appears that when completed, this system will function more like an expert system than an AI system, because of the limitations inherent in the development of all AI systems today. The technology is simply not yet available for a true AI system.

---

[21] B. G. Buchanan and E. H. Shortliffe, *Rule-Based Expert Systems: The MYCIN Experiments of the Stanford Heuristic Programming Project* (Reading, Mass.: Addison-Wesley Publishing Co., 1984), 4.

[22] S. Evans, "A Computer-Based Nursing Diagnosis Consultant," in *Proceedings of the Eighth Annual Symposium on Computer Applications in Medical Care*, ed. G. S. Cohen (Los Angeles: Institute of Electrical and Electronics Engineers Computer Society, 1984), 658–661.

[23] J. G. Ozbolt, "A Prototype Information System to Aid Nursing Decisions," in *Proceedings of the Sixth Annual Symposium on Computer Applications in Medical Care*, ed. B. I. Blum (Los Angeles: Institute of Electrical and Electronics Engineers Computer Society, 1982), 653–657; and J. G. Ozbolt et al., "Developing an Expert System for Nursing Practice," in *Proceedings of the Eighth Annual Symposium on Computer Applications in Medical Care*, 654–657.

CONCLUSION

The development of CADM systems is exciting to observe. Investigators are attempting to build data-base systems that have the ability to link isolated facts into comprehensive information that can be used to improve decision making. CADM systems help to transform data into information. Rose has written that before computers can become smarter, we need an explanation of how intelligence works in people.[24] Is the mind a formal symbol-manipulating system that the cognitive scientist will unravel?

Formal theory, which provides the basis for much of the current work on AI, postulates order in a seemingly random universe. Formal theory is based on induction, building knowledge from small, isolated pieces of information into rules and relationships. On the other hand, Dreyfus believes formalism leaves out situational properties such as opportunities, risks, and threats.[25] He calls for recognition of the primacy of intuition— learned responses based on previous experience. Benner has applied Dreyfus's work to nursing.[26] It remains to be seen if it will be possible to develop computer-assisted decision-making systems that have the properties of the human expert, such as reflection, language, ability to learn, ability to tolerate ambiguity, and so forth.

"Perhaps AI's most important applications will not be the programs that we write but the newfound ability to understand how people think."[27] Expert systems designed to improve clinical decision making places a reflecting mirror on these cognitive processes. This reflection may be changing our understanding of how we learn, think, and communicate. This reflection may also require nursing to examine the concepts within the nursing process and nursing diagnosis. Nursing has adopted CADM support systems that support management problem solving in health care settings today. Two CADM expert systems have been identified within nursing that are in different developmental stages and hold promise for the future. The impact of AI systems for improving nursing practice awaits further research and development.

---

[24] F. Rose, "The Black Knight of AI," *Science 85* (March 1985): 46–51.

[25] H. L. Dreyfus, "Holism and Hermeneutics," *Review of Metaphysics* 34 (1985): 3–24.

[26] Benner, *From Novice to Expert.*

[27] R. Schank and L. Hunter, "Artificial Intelligence: The Quest to Understand Thinking," *Byte* 10, no. 4 (1985): 155.

role

FACULTY PRACTICE: MAKING IT WORK

MARIANNE RONCOLI, PhD, RN
Robert Wood Johnson Clinical Nurse Scholar
School of Nursing
University of Pennsylvania
Philadelphia, Pennsylvania

Faculty practice is currently the most fashionable professional nursing practical role. A nurse engaged in faculty practice implements in the service setting the knowledge created and transmitted in the academic environment for the betterment of patients. Ford and Kitzman define it as practice "where activities related to patients have a scholarly orientation with associated scholarship outcomes and where the care of patients is the central focus."[1] Faculty practice is not merely designed to bring together antagonistic, argumentative, ornery factions in nursing; nor is it designed to provide "supernurse" role models for students; nor to enable faculty to feel the curriculum they have slaved over for years is relevant to the real world. Rather, the real goal of faculty practice, as Fagin has indicated, is power—power to influence patients and students, power to change health care delivery.[2]

Views expressed in this article are those of the author and no official endorsement of the Robert Wood Johnson Foundation is intended or should be inferred.

[1] Loretta Ford and Harriet J. Kitzman, "Organizational Perspectives on Faculty Practice: Issues and Challenges," in *Structure to Outcome: Making it Work*, ed. Kathryn E. Barnard, Proceedings of the First Annual Symposium on Nursing Faculty Practice (Kansas City, Mo.: American Academy of Nursing, December 1983).

[2] Claire Fagin, Keynote Address, American Academy of Nursing Second Faculty Practice Symposium, Phoenix, Arizona, January 24, 1985.

TYPES OF FACULTY PRACTICE

Diers has categorized various ways in which faculty can practice.[3] The first model is *joint appointments*, in which the administrations of service and academic institutions work out arrangements with faculty in schools of nursing and nurses in hospitals or other health care agencies to share the work of providing service to patients and education to students. The institutions must share a common philosophy that both students and patients will benefit from this arrangement.

Nurses may hold a joint appointment in only one institution with one central administration and one budget, including allocations for service and education. The University of Rochester exemplifies this model, in which there is no clear distinction between the clinicians and the educators. The clinical nursing chiefs of each department, including medicine, surgery, obstetrics, and so forth, are responsible for all patient care, teaching, and research. Clinical specialists (Clinicians II) are most likely to be directly teaching, as they negotiate a percentage of their time in either practice or education and are paid accordingly out of allocations in the combined university and Strong Memorial Hospital service budget.

A similar arrangement exists at Rush–Presbyteran–St. Luke's Medical Center in Chicago, where a matrix organizational structure allows practitioner-teachers to supervise the teaching of students and participate in the care of patients. These practitioner-teachers answer to department chairpersons and program directors who are responsible for both the patients' care and the students' instruction.

Joint appointments may also be arranged in two closely related institutions with two separate administrations with separate budgets. The most celebrated example of this type of joint appointment may be Case Western Reserve University in Cleveland. However, many schools and medical centers across the country use faculty practice models that resemble this system. Labels such as *collaboration* and *partnership* are used to describe these systems. The term *unification* is reserved for combined systems like Rush and Rochester.

Organizations operating from a collaborative or partnership framework provide more role options than that of the clinician-educator or Clinician II. Case Western Reserve has a separate administration for nursing service in the University Hospitals of Cleveland and in the university itself. Faculty may have an appointment in the University Hospital as an associate in nursing, where they have practice and research opportunities in the clinical areas along with their primary teaching responsibilities.

---

[3] Donna Diers, "Faculty Practice: Models, Methods and Madness," in *Cognitive Dissonance: Interpreting and Implementing Faculty Practice Roles in Nursing Education* (New York: National League for Nursing, 1980), 7–15.

Nurses in clinical agencies have clinical appointments in the school of nursing. Finally, faculty and staff may have shared appointments, in which each nurse negotiates a percentage of time and workload with the hospital and the school.[4] Variations of this model appear in other settings. The University of Arizona has made arrangements with Veterans Administration hospitals, and Beth Israel in Boston has developed collaborative arrangements with Boston University. Yale University, the University of Washington, and the University of Pennsylvania have developed faculty practice options, as have the University of Oklahoma and Stanford University Hospital Center.[5]

Another type of structure for faculty practice is a *dual appointment*, in which the individual basically holds two part-time jobs and is responsible to two separate administrators. The educational and service institutions have no formal or informal arrangement with each other. The faculty member, independently, arranges to teach in one institution and practice in another.

Another form of faculty practice is *independent practice*, where the school of nursing develops its own practice setting to provide service to clients, learning opportunities for students, and research subjects and researchable problems for nurse investigators. The most notable of these is the Nursing Consultation Center at Pennsylvania State University.[6] The center, which is managed by nurses, provides a place where individuals and families are cared for and encouraged to make life-style modifications in the face of developmental and situational life crisis, helped to cope with stress and change, and assisted in living with chronic illness. The center also provides blood pressure screening and monitoring and guidance and support in implementing selected treatment plans prescribed by physicians. Pace University, Adelphi University, and the City University of New York have developed informal nursing clinics providing similar services in community health agencies. Ongoing financial support and reimbursement mechanisms, however, have been extremely inadequate to date.

Finally, in addition to full-time teaching positions, faculty practice by *moonlighting*. It is interesting to note that in a national study of faculty practice, Anderson and Pierson found that "moonlighting," with little or no compensation, was the most frequently reported way faculty prac-

---

[4] Rosella M. Schlotfeldt and Jannetta MacPhail, "An Experiment in Nursing: Rationale and Characteristics," *American Journal of Nursing* 69 (1969): 1018–1023.

[5] Dorothy D. Nayer, "Unification: Bringing Nursing Service and Nursing Education Together," *American Journal of Nursing* 80 (June 1980): 1110–1114; Jo Frazer, "Future Perspectives for Faculty Practice—Credibility, Visibility, Accountability," in *Cognitive Dissonance*, 43–48; and Duane D. Walker, "Nursing Education and Service: The Payoffs of Partnership," *Nursing & Health Care* 6 (April 1985): 189–191.

[6] Janet A. Williamson, "Faculty Practice in a Nursing Center: An Integrated Model," in *Cognitive Dissonance*, 17–20.

ticed.[7] The sample, composed of primarily junior faculty without doctoral preparation or tenure, admittedly valued nursing practice; but the school offered neither a structure in which they could provide nursing service nor a faculty development program to enable them to create a vehicle for service delivery.

If faculty members are expressing a desire to practice, why then are so few teaching institutions providing the structure in which they can do so? The centers where unification and collaboration exist claim impressive outcomes: master teachers are available to students; the quality of nursing care improves; staff development costs are reduced as job commitment increases and attrition decreases; and students are better prepared to face the real world of nursing practice.[8] Why are these structures not easily replicated? Before existing systems can change, three problems need to be addressed: the distribution of *power*, *functions*, and *rewards*.

DISTRIBUTION OF POWER

Although power is, as Fagin suggests, the ultimate goal of partnership or unification, individuals may either gain or lose power when a system is initiated.[9] For example, if the positions of vice president for nursing affairs and the dean of the school of nursing are to be combined, which of the current occupants will fill the combined position? Similarly, if the positions of chairperson in the departments of nursing service and education are be unified, are either or both of the occupants of these positions equipped to handle the unified job? Someone will be out of a job completely, demoted, or made subordinate to a colleague with whom he or she is accustomed to relating as a peer. A typical solution to the problem has been to keep the department heads in their respective jobs and create another management level to which both chairpersons will answer. In an age of cost-containment, both hospitals and schools are reluctant to add another expensive management position to an already top-heavy bureaucracy. Unification can be a zero-sum game in which some people win and others lose.

For a combined system to work, individual power within a system will have to be subordinated to the overall professional power nursing would gain in the service of health care delivery and teaching effectiveness.

---

[7] Evelyn R. Anderson and P. Pierson, "An Explanatory Study of Faculty Practice: Views of Those Faculty Engaged in Practice Who Teach in an NLN-Accredited Baccalaureate Program," *Western Journal of Nursing Research* 5 (1983): 129–143.

[8] Judith Jezek, "Economic Realities of Faculty Practice," in *Cognitive Dissonance*, 37–41.

[9] Fagin, *op. cit.*

The architects of the plan need to remind themselves of why, in the words of Fagin and Diers, intelligent, educated people become nurses; namely, for

> a feeling of satisfaction derived from the caring role, indifference to power for its own sake, the recognition that one is a doer who enjoys doing for and with others, . . . and the pleasure associated with helping others from the position of peer rather than from the assumed superordinate position of some other professions.[10]

Nursing faculty and nursing staff have to refine negotiating skills, make trade-offs, and construct a vision of the mission before them. Deans, directors, department heads, and faculty need to remind themselves that protecting individual turf wins the battle of personal power but loses the war waged between nursing interests and those of other less patient- or student-oriented forces in the health care system.

The redistribution of power in a collaborative system will mean that no one's position is sacred or untouchable. Everyone's job will change. Faculty members may find themselves with less self-directed schedules, but more influence in the area of patient care. Staff nurses may have to expend more intellectual energy, but may get release time from routine tasks to go to the library to prepare a student seminar. People in administrative positions will have to teach faculty and practitioners the art of compromise.

DISTRIBUTION OF FUNCTIONS

When trade-offs are being contemplated, what work is to be divided up and how will it be done? How will people do practice, education, and research?

Like medicine, when nursing sought to upgrade professional practice, it moved the teaching of nursing into an academic setting. When Johns Hopkins established the first graduate program in medical education, the purpose was to "create a medical school environment where medicine was not only taught but studied."[11] Thus, a strong emphasis was established on research into medical practice. When nursing reforms elevated nursing education into academia, however, the university school of nursing became a place where nursing was taught and where the teaching—

---

[10] Claire Fagin and Donna Diers, "Nursing as Metaphor," *New England Journal of Medicine* 309 (July 14, 1983): 116.

[11] Rosemary Stevens, *American Medicine and the Public Interest* (New Haven: Yale University Press, 1971).

not the practice—of nursing was studied. Nursing, then, has a tradition of educational not clinical scholarship. As Smith and Christy have pointed out, we were still left with a dearth of master teachers.[12] The most knowledgeable clinicians, the most scholarly, educated nurses were not practicing or teaching nursing. No wonder Jeannette Spero at the University of Cincinnati, Judith Jezek at Rush–Presbyterian–St. Luke's Medical Center, Claire Fagin at the University of Pennsylvania, and Donna Diers at Yale University have advised diverting energy and resources into changing health care delivery, not nursing school curricula, and devising patient care interventions instead of teaching-learning strategies.[13]

Curriculum reform is about as popular as the miniskirt and teased hair. However, nursing's tradition of educational scholarship gives nurse educators reason to pause before embracing a collaborative or unification model that blends the functions of education with practice and research. They offer educationally sound objections to the unification model that the medical profession uses. Florence Nightingale's first school of nursing was an autonomous school that used St. Thomas Hospital as a clinical site. A colleague at the University of Pennsylvania and a recipient of the university's prestigious Lindback award for outstanding teaching, commenting on joint appointments, said; "I already have one job I can't finish; if I had a joint appointment, I would have two jobs I can't finish."

There are objections to unification within the medical profession itself. Heyssell states that the roles of teacher and practitioner in medical education are more distinct than they are alike.[14] Charns, Lawrence, and Weisbord conducted a study of professionals with multiple functions in academic medical centers and found that there were greater differences in the functions involved in practice, education, and research than there were among specialty groups.[15] For example, there were greater differences between practicing pediatric medicine and teaching pediatric medicine than between practicing pediatric medicine and practicing adult medicine or teaching pediatric medicine and teaching adult medicine. Furthermore, the professionals who were functioning in these varied roles underestimated the distinctions, resulting in a blurring of roles.

Examples of the blurring of roles appear daily in teaching hospitals. Consider, for example, the classic scene in which the medical professor

[12] Dorothy M. Smith, "Nursing Education and Nursing Service: A Dual or Separate Administrative Responsibility?" *Journal of the American Medical Association* 191 (1965): 144–146; and Teresa E. Christy, "Clinical Practice as a Function of Nursing Education: An Historical Analysis," *Nursing Outlook* 8 (1980):493–497.

[13] Jeannette Spero, "Faculty Practice as one Component of the Faculty Role," in *Cognitive Dissonance*, 1–6; Jezek, *op. cit.*, Fagin, *op. cit.*; and Diers, *op. cit.*

[14] Robert M. Heyssel, "The Challenge of Governance: The Relationship of the Teaching Hospital to the University," *Journal of Medical Education* 59 (1984): 162–168.

[15] Martin P. Charns, Paul R. Lawrence, and Marvin R. Weisbord, "Organizing Multiple Function Professionals in Academic Medical Centers," *TIMS Studies in Management Sciences* 5, (1977): 71–88.

makes rounds with the medical students and discusses the patient's "case" in front of the patient, whose anxiety is escalating. The students' attention is riveted on the professor, who is totally oblivious to the patient's distress. The physician is not only oblivious to the patient, he or she is oblivious to the conflicts inherent in combining the role of teacher and practitioner.[16]

The roles of teacher and researcher can be blurred as well. Departments of medicine in academic medical centers have the most renowned, accomplished researchers responsible for the medical education, practice, and research in their departments. They have reached their level of scientific prominence because they have developed sophisticated research teams in an environment where fledgling young medical scientists can freely explore new ideas with minimal supervision. However, when these famous researchers supervise the basic medical education of students and the medical care of patients with the same laissez-faire style they use in the laboratory, neither the medical student nor the patient benefits. The teaching hospital begins to resemble a large Montessori school for medical education, where students are allowed to roam through the corridors unsupervised, familiarizing themselves with the exigencies of patient care. These researchers may be famous, but they have underestimated the complexity of combining the roles of educator, practitioner, and researcher.

I would propose that this system works as well as it does because a single-function professional—the nurse—is primarily concerned with patient care. The nurse wards off disaster, protects the patient, and provides medical instruction to the student physicians. The breakdown in communication between physician and nurses is directly related to the fact that nurses are primarily concerned with patient care, while the physicians are addressing an agenda of research, teaching, and, often, private business as well. If nurses assumed multiple functions along with the physicians, they might well begin to appreciate the complexity of the physician's role and relate in a more collegial way. Does nursing really want to embrace this multiple-function model the way medicine has? Sovie admits that one of the problems in the unification system is overwork and burnout.[17] Perhaps, because of their educational sophistication, nurse faculty and nursing staff appreciate the complexity of the roles, but attempt to accomplish them anyway, albeit unsatisfactorily, because medicine has set the standard.

Charns, Lawrence, and Weisbord suggest that one way out of this untenable situation is to develop a matrix organizational structure, where

---

[16] *Ibid.*

[17] Margaret D. Sovie, "Unifying Education and Practice: One Medical Center's Design, Parts I and II," *Journal of Nursing Administration* 11 (1981): 41–49, 30–32.

the functions of practice, education, and research within each departmental specialty are organized separately and distinctly.[18] As illustrated in Figure 1, educators (E), practitioners (P) and researchers (R) are responsible to *both* the chairperson of specialty departments and the director of the specific programs in which these multiple-function professionals are involved. If one is involved in both education and practice, one is responsible to each of the directors of the respective education or practice programs as well as to the chairperson of one's specialty department. This structure not only preserves the distinction of functions, but also delineates the responsibilities of each program and specialty. In this setting, role conflicts can be addressed and realistic work assignments can be devised that will not compromise function performance.

This structure is already in operation at Rush–Presbyterian–St. Luke's Medical Center (see Figure 2). Both chairpersons of specialty departments and program directors have line authority and interact with each other in the business of education, practice, and research. Why then is this system not easily replicated? Fagin concludes that a matrix nursing organization is only one system within the complex structure—a single bureaucratic slice within a multidimensional medical center.[19] Moreover, each academic medical center is unique and complex in its own way. Whatever nursing organization is developed, then, must fit into the existing organizational design; no one model will work everywhere. Furthermore, if the functions of education, practice, and research are indeed distinct, they must be supervised, evaluated, rewarded, and organized separately. It is the functions, then, not the structure that must be addressed when unification is contemplated.

DISTRIBUTION OF REWARDS

The final problem preventing more faculty from practicing is the inadequacy of rewards. Faculty have not only not been rewarded for faculty practice, they have been penalized. The rewards traditionally available in academia—tenure and promotion—are difficult or impossible to obtain. If a structure is in place that clearly distinguishes between the functions of education, practice, and research, tenure and promotion should *not* be rewards for faculty practice. The problem becomes not how to reward faculty practice, but how to reward advanced nursing practice itself, within a unification or collaboration system.

The University of Rochester, the University of Pennsylvania and others have experimented with different faculty classifications, including tradi-

---

[18] Charns, Lawrence, and Weisbord, "Organizing Multiple Function Professionals in Academic Medical Centers."

[19] Fagin, *op. cit.*

Figure 1. Matrix Organizational Structure for Education, Practice, and Research

Matrix Organizational Structure

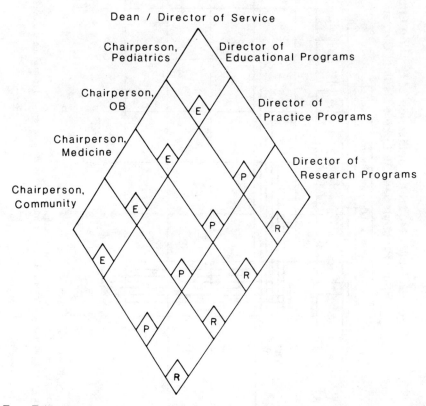

E = Educators
P = Practitioners
R = Researchers

Adapted from: Martin P. Charns, Paul R. Lawrence, and Marvin R. Weisbord, "Organizing Multiple Function Professionals in Academic Medical Centers," *TIMS Studies in Management Sciences* 5 (1977): 71–78.

Figure 2. Matrix Model for Unification of Nursing Effort at Rush–Presbyterian–St. Luke's Medical Center

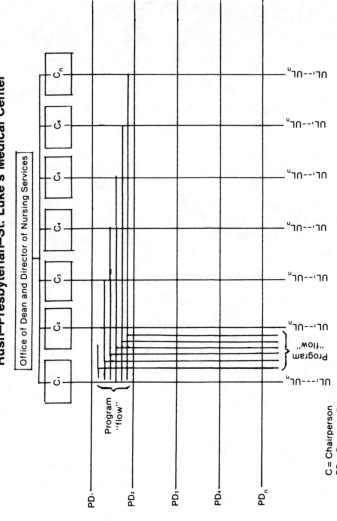

C = Chairperson
PD = Program Director (education/service/research)
UL = Unit Leader (Each department has as many unit leaders as required to manage the workload.)

Source: Luther Christman, "The Practitioner Teacher," *Nurse Educator* 4 (1979): 10.

tional tenure-track positions, clinical non-tenure-track positions, and tenure-track positions that provide additional time in which to qualify.[20] In the non-tenure- or extended-tenure-track positions, however, the rewards can amount to little more than eliminating or delaying the stress of a tenure decision. As Holm candidly states, being a credible practitioner-teacher is a reward that becomes less and less important with time.[21] After a while resentment builds up. Why should nursing faculty spend all their effort practicing nursing, when their faculty colleagues receive the same salary, benefits, and promotions without leaving the safety of their offices?

Several writers have addressed this issue, describing systems of faculty practice compensation plans similar to those developed by medicine.[22] The faculty member receives a standard base salary according to rank, plus an augmented salary based on funds generated through practice—generally through third-party reimbursement. In large medical centers, third-party reimbursement is not currently possible since nursing care, unlike medical care, is not reimbursed on a fee-for-service basis. With more and more states providing third-party reimbursement for advanced levels of nursing practice, however, it is necessary to determine how feasible and economical it is to bill, collect, and disburse reimbursements from third-party payers. Moreover, nurses may not have the same incentives to join practice plans as physicians do. Often these practice plans provide office space, equipment, and malpractice insurance more cheaply than the physicians can provide for themselves. Nurses, especially psychiatric nurses, may find themselves better off "moonlighting" or taking a dual appointment that includes an adjunct faculty position and an independent private practice, because it is more profitable and less troublesome to practice this way. A faculty practice plan would have to be attractive enough not to jeopardize the financial reward system that independent nurse practitioners have fought so courageously to win. Status, influence, patient referral systems, and a public relations system advertising nursing services to the community would lure nurse practitioners into an academic environment where their expertise could be shared with students and nurse investigators. These practice plans should also address free-standing nursing clinics where financial support is almost non-existent.

---

[20] Nancy A. Kent, "Evaluating the Practice Component for Faculty Rank and Tenure," in *Cognitive Dissonance*, 21–26.

[21] Karyn Holm, "Faculty Practice—Noble Intentions Gone Awry?" *Nursing Outlook* 29 (1981): 655–657.

[22] Linda Aiken, ed., *Health Policy and Nursing Practice* (New York: McGraw-Hill Book Co., 1981); Shirley S. Chater, "Faculty Practice Considerations in Academic Health Centers' Schools of Nursing," in *Structure to Outcome*; and Connie Curran and Donovan W. Riley, "Faculty Practice Plans: Will They Work for Nurses?" *Nursing Economics* 2 (1984): 319–324.

THE IDEAL FACULTY PRACTICE ENVIRONMENT

The ideal setting for faculty practice resembles a company in the extremely competitive, rapidly changing high-technology field.[23] For example, the president of the successful and highly profitable Intel Corporation attributes his company's ability to maintain a competitive edge in the fast-paced industry that manufactures silicon chips for computers to the egalitarian, informal work environments he and other high-technology executives create.[24] They have little interest in executive dining rooms, reserved parking spaces, or first-class airline accommodations. Rather than plush private offices, the presidents, boards of directors, and engineers all work in functional private cubicles designed to develop ideas, not corporate images. There is, as Grove says, little divergence between the people in *power* and the people with *knowledge*. In an explosive industry where changes occur daily, high-technology firms cannot afford to wait for the knowledge to reach the boss and the boss to become familiar with it. The boss has to be down on the ground floor of research and development, not up in the executive tower of corporate decision-making. The boss has to be involved in engineering, marketing, production, public relations—in short, every aspect of the business—if he or she is to keep pace with competitors. Moreover, the employees in close proximity to the managers participate in the decision-making process.

This environment can exist on any given nursing care unit—an intensive care unit, a cooperative care unit, a step-down unit, an outpatient clinic, or a freestanding nursing clinic. The people with *power*, the administrators of nursing and medical care, work side by side with the people with *knowledge*, the educators and researchers. They would all share common goals—for example, the submission of a grant to study a patient feeding problem, a workable discharge program for the Smith family, or a publication on a retrospective chart review.

The analogy between a small high-technology firm that may have evolved from the back of someone's garage or basement and a complex academic medical center may seem ludicrous. However, if some kind of matrix organizational structure is in place, small decentralized units can exist in which the staff functions independently, autonomously, and with a great deal of accountability. Faculty and researchers should only practice and do research in units where the patient care coordinator or head nurse has the authority and responsibility for nursing staff and nursing care. Primary nursing should be in operation, and levels of nursing prac-

---

[23] Marianne Roncoli, "Nursing in Silicon Valley," *Research Quarterly* (Center for Nursing Research, University of Pennsylvania) 14 (1984): 1–2.

[24] Andrew S. Grove, "Breaking the Chains of Command," *Newsweek*, October 3, 1983, 23.

tice should be evident so that functions of and rewards for education, practice, and research can be delineated. A nurse educator or researcher could fit in easily by negotiating time and responsibilities with the staff. In a decentralized, autonomous unit, the *functions* of patient care, research, and teaching can evolve into manageable roles. This should be the home base for a clinical researcher—an egalitarian, informal setting where collegial relationships between people can grow.

STRATEGIES FOR FACULTY PRACTICE

Several nurses involved in or contemplating joint appointments have suggested strategies for implementation. One nursing administrator devised a reciprocity agreement for faculty, enabling them to negotiate a role for themselves in the clinical setting.[25] Like the mechanisms discussed by Ford and Kitzman, including contracts, letters of agreement, exchange of service mechanisms, consortium arrangements, it need not necessarily involve the deans and directors of nursing service.[26] Again, if units are really autonomous, faculty should be able to work out these relationships and agreements with the unit staff and put an overall approval and compensation plan in place.

Someone on an administrative level, however, should coordinate the efforts including, as Blazeck and colleagues suggest, the publication of joint faculty and school calendars, newsletters, and departmental communications.[27] Some enterprising systems analyst might also want to obtain a Ford Foundation grant to study why it takes three weeks for a memo in the school to reach its destination in the hospital. A faculty or staff person might also want to experiment with a full-time teaching, service, or research appointment. A scholar-in-residence or a practitioner-in-residence program should be available.

Finally, all the experts on faculty practice agree that the most essential ingredient for a successful collaborative effort is the support of colleagues and administrators. People who want to practice need to do so in an environment where the professional nurses share the philosophy that practice is not merely an interesting option but a professional necessity. If nurses do not have this support, they should move on. They should examine the roster of deans who signed the Statement of Belief Regarding Faculty Practice that appeared in nursing magazines, pick one or two in

---

[25] Tamar Gilson-Parkevich, "Stepchildren in the Family: Aiming Toward Synergy Between Nursing Education and Service—From the Nursing Service Perspective," in *Structure to Outcome.*

[26] Ford and Kitzman, "Organizational Perspectives on Faculty Practice."

[27] Alice Maus Blazeck et al., "Unification: Nursing Education and Nursing Practice," *Nursing & Health Care* 3 (January 1982): 18–24.

desirable locations, and give them a call.[28] They are looking for a critical mass of clinical scholars who believe that those who can do—and those who do very well, teach!

BIBLIOGRAPHY

Bracken, R., and Christman, L. "An Incentive Program Designed to Reward Clinical Competence." *Journal of Nursing Administration* 10 (1978): 8–18.

Collison, Carol R., and Mary Ann Parson. "Is Practice a Viable Faculty Role?" *Nursing Outlook* 28(1980): 677–679.

Curtis, Marcia. "Evaluating the Clinical Performance of Faculty: Fact or Fantasy." In *Cognitive Dissonance: Interpreting and Implementing Faculty Practice Roles in Nursing Education*, 27–32. New York: National League for Nursing, 1980.

Engstrom, Janet L. "University, Agency, and Collaborative Models for Nursing Research." *Image: The Journal of Nursing Scholarship* 16(1984): 76–80.

MacPhail, Janetta. "Promoting Collaboration/Unification Models for Nursing Education and Service." In *Cognitive Dissonance: Interpreting and Implementing Faculty Practice Roles in Nursing Education*, 33–36. New York: National League for Nursing, 1980.

Pierik, Madaline M. "Joint Appointments: Collaboration for Better Patient Care." *Nursing Outlook* 21(1973):576–579.

Schlotfeldt, Rosella M., and Jannetta MacPhail. "An Experiment in Nursing: Introducing Planned Change." *American Journal of Nursing* 69(1969): 1247–1251.

———. An Experiment in Nursing: Implementing Planned Change. *American Journal of Nursing* 69(1969): 1475–1480.

---

[28] "Statement of Belief Regarding Faculty Practice," *Nurse Educator* 4 (1979): 5.

JOINT NURSING APPOINTMENTS— A MEANS TO AN END

JOAN FARRELL BROWNIE, RN, PhD
Dean and Professor, School of Nursing
Medical College of Virginia
Virginia Commonwealth University
Associate Director of Nursing Administration
Medical College of Virginia Hospitals
Richmond, Virginia

Joint appointments in nursing are frequently praised or criticized without attention to the underlying organizational structure that they serve and the mission of the agencies concerned. Joint appointments may be made in name only or based on unrealistic expectations. They may be made with shared fiscal responsibility or without regard to budget commitments. They may be made with superficial cause to satisfy philosophical problems in service and education, or they may be made with serious intent to improve nursing education and patient care services.

Generalization about joint appointments will not help nursing improve clinical nursing programs. Nevertheless, some basic points should be seriously considered. The success of such appointments depends on the commitment of the cooperating parties, the ability to support the concept fiscally, and the expertise of the individuals carrying out the joint roles. All three factors must be present if the concept and practice are to succeed.

At Medical College of Virginia (MCV), Virginia Commonwealth University, there is a real interest in joint appointments and a growing commitment to making this concept work. All parties are fully aware, however, that the joint appointments are only a *means to an end*. At the MCV Health Science Center, our philosophy supports quality education in all professional schools and the best possible patient care for the patients at MCV Hospitals. Quality instruction in managing clinical nursing problems cannot take place without access to a variety of appropriate clinical environments and to patients with a diversity of problems. Faculty must teach and practice according to current nursing concepts and investigate nursing problems using valid research approaches. Opportunities for nursing education and nursing research depend on legitimate access to patients. The joint appointment is *one* way for nursing faculty to gain this access. Joint appointments also give nursing faculty influence in matters of patient care and allow them to make decisions concerning the quality of care provided in the institution. At MCV, all professional schools and their faculty are concerned with and committed to quality patient care as well as quality in educational experiences.

Professional nursing education programs that take place in a university health science center are unique because of their access to an academic environment of research and practice unlike that of most other higher degree nursing programs. At MCV, this uniqueness is exemplified by the association of nursing with the School of Basic Science and four other health professional schools—the Schools of Medicine, Dentistry, Pharmacy, and Allied Health Professions—as well as with a vast hospital and clinic system. The MCV hospital system is responsive to the urban health care needs of the city, to the state's needs for tertiary referral services, and to national needs for basic and applied research.

Because preparation for professional nursing practice requires emphasis on scientific theory and clinical experience, a nursing school such as MCV with a hospital as part of the system has opportunities and responsibilities far beyond those of schools that find it necessary to contract out for practice experiences. The opportunities lie in the chance to work closely with colleagues from a variety of disciplines, to select learning experiences from a wide range of clinical services, and to gain an awareness of the organization and operation of a large health service facility. On the other hand, the responsibilities include a commitment to the prudent use of clinical resources with thoughtful attention to the quality and the ethics of patient care and clinical research.

COLLABORATIVE MODEL

In the complex environment of a nursing school in a university health science center, a collaborative model for nursing service and education provides the direction for integrating the activities and services provided by Nursing Service and the School of Nursing. The collaborative model refers to a system in which the MCV Hospitals Nursing Service staff and the faculty of the MCV School of Nursing work actively together on matters concerning academic excellence in nursing at the Virginia Commonwealth University (see Figure 1). The basis on which the collaborative model is being built is the "Statement on Nursing Education and Practice in a University Health Science Center," which I developed as dean of nursing and associate director of nursing administration at MCV, together with the director of nurses.

Academic excellence can only be achieved in an environment dedicated to excellence in clinical practice. Consequently, issues addressed in this model include the quality of patient care, the education of nursing students seeking baccalaureate and advanced degrees, and continuing studies for staff nurses, nursing administrators, and faculty. Because many aspects of nursing education dealing with patient care require systematic inquiry to explicate problems of interest, research is also viewed as an integral component of the collaborative model.

The model's purpose is to identify ways and means by which nursing faculty, nursing service administrators, and clinical specialists or unit leaders can work collaboratively for excellence in clinical practice through quality patient care, sound educational programming for graduate and undergraduate students, and continuing studies for staff nurses, nursing administrators, and faculty. The four substantive areas of collaboration in the model are practice, education, research, and administration. The joint appointment can be used as a means of carrying out all of the collaborative roles at all levels.

The unifying objective of the model is excellent patient care. Additional objectives follow from this. The collaborative model is expected to:

1. Increase faculty presence and influence within the patient care environment.
2. Provide for nursing service input into curriculum planning.
3. Strengthen particular course content in both the formal curriculum and in continuing education through input from service regarding current practice modes and input from education regarding the theoretical bases of content.
4. Enhance joint research activity by providing accessibility to research populations and identifying clinical problems to be studied; sharing knowledge of research designs for studying clinical problems; and utilizing research findings in practice environments.
5. Provide a structure within which education and service leaders can jointly address issues facing health care.
6. Unify the voice of nursing within the university community.

Structurally, the model is designed to ensure collaboration and predictability in relationships between school and hospital from the level of

Figure 1. Collaborative Model of Education/Service Relationships

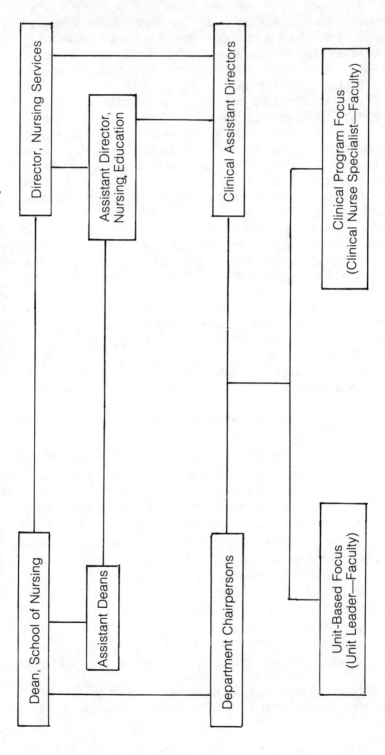

the unit leader and faculty through the levels of the assistant director and chairperson, and the director and dean. The linkages are tailored to maximize use of the existing structure of each organization. Commitments are reciprocal; they are designed to be negotiated for feasibility with one's immediate superior and evaluated annually.

Ideally, individual faculty members will be assigned consistently to one hospital unit and will be participating members of unit activities and decisions. Likewise, unit coordinators will participate directly and indirectly in the teaching of students. In each case, faculty and unit coordinators will function as advocates for the other. Similarly, assistant directors and chairpersons will serve as consultants to each other, will contribute to the accomplishment of planning and programming missions of service and education, will teach and supervise as appropriate, and will communicate on a regular basis.

STRUCTURE FOR COLLABORATION

The relationships between school and hospital personnel can be structured and actualized in a variety of ways. The following sections describe each component of the proposed structure of relationships within the collaborative model illustrated in Figure 1.

Assistant Deans and the Assistant Director of Nursing Education

The assistant deans coordinate with the assistant director of nursing education. The areas of joint responsibility and collaboration for the assistant dean for clinical affairs and resource development and the assistant director of nursing education are the following:

1. Coordinate clinical rotations for undergraduate students.
2. Coordinate jointly sponsored continuing education activities.
3. Maintain records of faculty practice arrangements.
4. Process clinical associate applications and maintain clinical associate appointment contracts.
5. Collaborate in developing and implementing work-study arrangements.
6. Communicate changes in clinical practice expectations for students.

The assistant dean for academic affairs and the assistant director of nursing education have the following joint responsibilities:

1. Communicate changes in undergraduate and graduate curricula that have implications for practice, as well as changes in the practice environment that affect education.

2. Maintain records of the clinical rotations of graduate students and preceptors.
3. Collaborate in developing and implementing educational research projects.

The assistant director of nursing education also serves as a member of the undergraduate curriculum committee.

In the area of clinical research, there is a need to develop linkages between the associate director for research and development, the research nurse, and the assistant dean for clinical affairs and resource development.

Department Chairperson and Assistant Director of Nursing

The reality of the current administrative organization of the school and hospital necessitates the development of a structure to assure the vital relationship between each clinical and educational department. The structure describes the relationship between departmental chairpersons and assistant directors of nursing, based on departmental, clinical, or administrative ties.

When the assistant director and department chairperson do not share a common clinical background or when numerous assistant directors are linked with one chairperson, the structure allows delegation of selected functions. In such cases, the relationship at the level of the department chairperson and assistant director facilitates conceptual and long-range planning, while the delegated activities have a more operational focus.

Within this structure, the chairperson is expected to:

1. Provide ongoing consultation to assistant director.
2. Provide clinical teaching, continuing education, precepting, supervising.
3. Serve on selected Nursing Service departmental committees and task forces.
4. Provide representation on departmental practice councils (can be delegated).

Expectations of the assistant director or associate director include the following:

1. Provide ongoing consultation to chairperson.
2. Make direct contributions to teaching and program development.
3. Serve on selected School of Nursing committees and task forces.

The following are joint responsibilities of the department chairperson and assistant director. Starred items may be delegated.

1. Schedule regular meetings at least quarterly.
2. Engage in strategic long-term planning (e.g., program planning).
3. Do facilities planning.
4. Exchange agendas and minutes.
5. Negotiate time of faculty, unit coordinator, and clinical specialist.
*6. Be involved in course planning, including continuing education.
*7. Collaborate in routine problem solving.
8. Collaborate in research and projects on an ongoing basis.
*9. Contribute expertise in departmental deliberations.
*10. Collaborate on special projects of short duration (3–4 months).
*11. Serve as resource on professional issues, such as certification.

Unit and Clinical Program Levels

Both the unit-based focus and the clinical program focus for collaboration are stratified based on Styles' unity continuum.[1] The three levels of collaboration for faculty, nursing unit leaders, and clinical specialists are communication, consultation, and consent. The levels are additive, in the sense that each builds on the last, incorporating the expectations of the previous level.

Unit-Based Focus. The unit-based construct has been developed for those faculty and nursing service unit leaders (unit coordinators, administrative clinician Bs, or clinicians) who desire a unit-based focus (see Table 1). Collaborative activities are directed toward clients in one clinical unit.

Clinical Program Focus. The clinical program focus construct was developed for faculty and clinical nurse specialists who desire a clinical focus unrelated to a particular clinical unit (see Table 2). This construct involves collaborative activities directed toward clients who may be on various units in different nursing services departments.

---

[1]Margretta M. Styles, "Reflections on Collaboration and Unification," *Image: The Journal of Nursing Scholarship* 16 (Winter 1984): 21–23.

Table 1. Unit-Based Focus Collaboration Model

Level	Time Commitment	Expectations of Faculty	Expectations of Unit Leader	Shared Expectations
I. Communication	4 hours or less per week	Familiarity with Nursing Service/unit hospital policies and procedures that influence unit/student practices.	Awareness of course objectives and objectives for clinical experience. Orientation of students to unit. Collaboration in making patient assignments for students.	Mutual interaction and sharing of patient care data. On-the-spot teaching. Observation and sharing of patterns of behavior affecting patient care. Positive response to students and staff on a daily basis. Mutual resource sharing and consultation (clinical, theoretical, administrative) on an ad hoc basis. Scheduled and spontaneous feedback sessions between unit leader and faculty to evaluate experience.
II. Consultation	Variable intensity—averages at least 4 hours per week	Interface with leadership team members when appropriate.	Awareness of course objectives in relation to overall curriculum.	Mutual interaction and sharing of patient care data through established unit systems (care planning, patient care conferences, shift report, student conferences).

III. Consent	Sustained contact—averages 8–16 hours per week	Engaging in direct practice on unit by role modeling clinical skills and by applying nursing theory. Participation in unit staff meetings and committees as appropriate.	Consultation as complex situations arise (patient care, unit mangement).	Unit acceptance of students as integral part of unit (e.g., knows students by name and skill level).	Rounds with students and staff on selected patients. Formal teaching exchanges (individual and group learning endeavors). Collaboration on special projects of short duration (research, writing, educational materials). Identification of questions for further study or research.
		Teaching and/or mentoring students in the clinical area.			Continuing collaboration in problem-solving in complex patient situations and unit management. Ongoing, active sharing of resources. Collaboration on student learning issues. Ongoing collaboration on research (planning, implementing, evaluating).

Table 2. Clinical Program Focus Collaboration Model

Level	Time Commitment	Expectations of Faculty	Expectations of Clinical Nurse Specialist	Shared Expectations
I. Communication	4 hours or less per week	Awareness of hospital clinical nurse specialist with similar area of expertise.	Awareness of School of Nursing faculty with similar area of expertise.	Communication regarding area of interest. Sharing of resources and knowledge. Casual, occasional interaction regarding educational needs and concerns.
II. Consultation	Variable intensity—averages at least 4 hours per week	Participation in continuing education and/or inservice activities for Nursing Service personnel. Possible negotiation of a selectively chosen caseload of a limited number of patients.	Participation in classes in the School of Nursing. Willing and positive precepting of students.	Collaboration on special projects (such as nursing diagnosis) for patients with complex problems. (Individuals collaborating at this level would hold a clinical associate appointment with either the School of Nursing or Nursing Service as appropriate.)

| III. Consent | Sustained contact—averages 8–16 hours per week | Maintainence of limited case-load of patients in area of speciality. Demonstration of practitioner/teacher role activities in school and hospital.* | Regular, planned formal teaching activities. Participation in course planning in areas of specialty. | Collaboration on a clinical research project. Collaboration with staff on various units for ongoing problem solving of complex patient situations. (Individuals performing at this level have either a formalized joint appointment between the School and Nursing Services, or a negotiated reciprocal agreement.) |

*See Luther Christman, "The Practitioner/Teacher: A Working Paper for Faculty at Rush University College of Nursing and Allied Health Sciences," in *The Practitioner-Teacher Role: Practice What You Teach*, ed. L. Machan (Wakefield, Mass.: Nursing Resources, 1980), 5–8.

CONCLUSION

Although nursing programs have moved away from hospital-based teaching, a significant amount of clinical content can and should be taught in a hospital environment. If a university owns and manages that hospital environment, there should be no reason not to work out joint arrangements that will benefit nursing education and nursing service. Joint appointments can be worked out with affiliates as well. The process probably will be a little more tedious, but it can be done if the three prerequisites mentioned earlier—commitment, financial support, and expertise—are available. For schools that are not part of a university or college that owns and operates a hospital, the process may be somewhat different.

Joint appointments may not be considered necessary, but as we face diminishing funds in both service and education, we in nursing education probably will have to pay for some or all of our clinical facilities. This may be in the form of outright monetary payments or it may be an exchange for service given by faculty and students. Joint appointments are one way that we in nursing education can capitalize on hospital funds to provide better patient care and better nursing education.

BIBLIOGRAPHY

Baker, C. M. "Moving Toward Interdependence: Strategies for Collaboration." *Journal of Nursing Administration* 11 (1981): 34–39.

Blazeck, Alice Maus, Janice Selekman, Mary Timpe, and Zane Robinson Wolf. "Unification: Nursing Education and Nursing Practice." *Nursing and Health Care* 3 (January 1982): 18–24.

Christman, Luther. "The Practitioner/Teacher: A Working Paper for Faculty at Rush University College of Nursing and Allied Health Sciences. In *The Practitioner-Teacher Role: Practice What You Teach*, ed. L. Machan, 5–8. Wakefield, Mass.: Nursing Resources, 1980.

Christy, Teresa E. "Clinical Practice as a Function of Nursing Education: An Historical Analysis." *Nursing Outlook* 28 (August 1980): 493–497.

Gresham, M. L. "Joint Appointments." In *The Clinical Nurse Specialist in Theory and Practice*, ed. A. B. Hamric and J. Spross, 129–148. New York: Grune & Stratton, 1983.

Holm, Karyn. "Faculty Practice—Noble Intentions Gone Awry? *Nursing Outlook* 29(1981): 655–657.

Smith, G. R. "Compensating Faculty for Their Clinical Practice." *Nursing Outlook* 28 (1980): 673–676.

Sovie, Margaret D. "Unifying Education and Practice: One Medical Center's Design, Part 1." *Journal of Nursing Administration* 11 (1981): 41–48.

―――. "Unifying Education and Practice: One Medical Center's Design, Part 2." *Journal of Nursing Administration* 11 (1981): 30–32.

Styles, Margretta M. "Reflections on Collaboration and Unification." *Image: The Journal of Nursing Scholarship* 16 (1984): 21–23.

―――. *Task Force on Education/Service Relationships Final Report.* Richmond: Medical College of Virginia, Virginia Commonwealth University, December 1984.

FULFILLING THE COMMITMENT TO PRACTICE WITHOUT JOINT FACULTY APPOINTMENTS

ERLINE P. McGRIFF, EdD, RN, FAAN
Professor, Division of Nursing
New York University
New York, New York

This paper focuses on improving nursing practice *without* joint faculty appointments. My thesis is that the mission of nursing education is to serve the student; the mission of nursing service is to serve the consumer public; and nursing education and nursing service meet *in practice*.

Joint faculty appointments are neither feasible nor desirable in every situation. Not every faculty member can or should embrace the concept of joint faculty appointments. Whatever system is used must be appropriate for the institution of which it is a part. There is no one answer or model that will serve as a panacea. Each situation must be examined and a determination made about which plan is most appropriate.

There are other ways besides joint practice for nursing to achieve its professional aims. Nursing education and nursing service can develop equitable institutional arrangements that will support the philosophy and objectives of both. Scientific inquiry that involves opportunities and options to identify problems; to study phenomena; to plan, implement, and test intervention; and to institute change to improve nursing and health care may be achieved without joint faculty appointments.

NURSING ROLES

The major roles in nursing are administration, teaching, research, and practice. Nursing must have control over each of these diverse areas, a situation that gives rise to many questions. How can nurses in each of these roles be structurally isolated from one another but still collaborate and cooperate effectively? Is it necessary to bring nursing service and nursing education under one administrative head to achieve this? How can nursing education be infused by the realities of clinical practice and nursing service injected with the enthusiasm of learners and the introduction of new nursing knowledge?[1] Must all nursing researchers engage in nursing practice to document outcomes of their research? Must the dean and all faculty members assume clinical responsibilities and demonstrate clinical competence as well as academic qualifications? Must part of teaching include "doing"? Must every faculty member be expected to take responsibility for the quality of nursing care in the clinical setting? Should clinicians assume teaching responsibilities? What system will be used for titling and appointing such persons to the faculty? What system of reimbursement will be used?

The administrative separation of nursing education from nursing service need not result in ineffective communication, coordination, and collaboration. Certainly, many nursing education programs in higher education have historically collaborated with nursing service to fulfill their mission. College and university schools not related to hospitals and those where hospitals did not exist or were located elsewhere have been primary examples of successful programs without joint faculty appointments. Close associations exist between the educational units in nursing and the nursing departments of health care agencies used for clinical learning experiences for both undergraduate and graduate nursing students and faculty.

Many resources other than traditional institutional settings are available for the selection of learning experiences. Selected instructional opportunities in such settings are essential, first for the student to relate theory to practice, and, second, to assist students in becoming socialized into the nursing profession. Does this mean that health care settings are dependent on educational institutions? The answer, quite properly, is "of course." But such dependence should not be for provision of services, as is the case in joint faculty appointments; rather it consists of the expectation that educational institutions will prepare graduates who will seek attractive careers in diverse health care settings and will become true professional colleagues providing excellent service, advancing knowl-

---

[1] Linda H. Aiken, ed., *Health Policy and Nursing Practice* (New York: McGraw-Hill Book Co., 1981).

edge, and influencing health policies.[2] This is where nursing education and nursing service will achieve their common endeavor and close the gap: *in the practice of nursing.* These nurses should fulfill a professional role and become models of competency that provide an exemplary learning climate for future nursing students.

The pressures of assuming responsibilities in both a nursing education program and an organized nursing service are tremendous, and both settings require a special kind of expertise. Socialization into each role is quite different. Challenges in providing nursing service and staffing are great and require ongoing attention. Equally demanding are the responsibilities for leadership in curriculum development and evaluation, student and faculty recruitment, and maintaining and enhancing high standards of nursing education. Why should it be necessary to have faculty members assume the additional responsibilities of practice for nursing to become a respected discipline that will contribute more effectively to the total care of the patient? Can the person with such a dual appointment really do justice to both?

No person should be placed in the position of serving two masters. Joel found that the "time divided between two systems does create strain and some wasted effort in shifting focus from one area to another."[3] When faculty with both teaching and service responsibilities must choose between the demands of nursing service and teaching, then service takes priority.

UNIVERSITY EXPECTATIONS

Universities seek faculty who will demonstrate excellence in teaching, research, and other scholarly endeavors and will render service to the institution, profession, and community. Practice per se has not been viewed as a credible vehicle for scholarship and has not weighed heavily in the formula for promotion and tenure.[4] Joint faculty appointments place additional pressures on faculty to meet university requirements for promotion and tenure. To what extent does the responsibility for the day-to-day operation of nursing services drain faculty members of energy necessary for the role of productive scholar they are expected to fulfill? Planned practice in the service setting, as an expected component of faculty

[2] Dorothy Nayer, "Unification: Bringing Nursing Service and Nursing Education Together," *American Journal of Nursing* 80 (June 1980): 1110–1114.

[3] Lucille A. Joel, "Stepchildren in the Family: Aiming Toward Synergy Between Nursing Education and Service—From the Faculty Perspective," in *Structure to Outcome: Making it Work,* ed. K. E. Barnard (Kansas City, Mo.: American Academy of Nursing, 1983), 43–57.

[4] A. Yarcheski and N. E. Mahon, "The Unification Model in Nursing: Risk-Receptivity Profiles Among Deans, Tenured, and Non-tenured Faculty in the United States," *Western Journal of Nursing Research* (in press).

responsibility, may also result in unrealistic and heavy workloads and schedules.

Faculty who are engaged in teaching, theory development, and research that will enhance the effectiveness of practice may desire access to clinical settings. Joint faculty appointments change the focus of responsibility for faculty members and should not be necessary for faculty members to have research and practice privileges. In a negotiated arrangement with a clinical setting, a faculty member might create or design and evaluate innovative practice roles or models for nursing; demonstrate ability to apply and test theory in practice settings; and serve as a role model for students and peers in professional practice and in the investigation of practice issues. Such contributions may well be given consideration for inclusion in the decision on promotion and tenure. In such a negotiated arrangement, both faculty and staff may be viewed as role models, each recognizing and respecting the other's competencies. In addition, they will serve as consultants to one another and may increase interdisciplinary involvement. Consultative services might relate to technical innovations, theories, research findings, program planning, and problem solving.

MAINTAINING CLINICAL COMPETENCE

No one would deny that faculty involved in the teaching of clinical nursing must be clinically competent in what they teach and must be able to convey their expertise to their students. The arguments arise over how such faculty can remain expert in their area without being overwhelmed by the other pressures of the academic community for research, publishing, and service.

How can nursing faculty avoid losing touch with the realities of nursing practice and losing credibility with students and colleagues? Certainly, faculty who are with students in clinical areas—usually on a weekly basis—are keeping in touch with reality. Various experiences and opportunities—other than joint appointments—are available to assist faculty members in maintaining and enhancing their clinical practice competency.

Faculty may seek employment in nursing service during summers and semester breaks or other free time for the purpose of maintaining and enhancing their clinical skills. Even though such a mechanism may be considered continuing education by some, such employment does serve the purpose of updating clinical skills.[5] Faculty appointments on a nine-

---

[5] M. V. Batey, "Structured Consideration for the Social Integration of Nursing," in *Structure to Outcome*, 1–11.

or ten-month basis provide free time for faculty to plan such activities. Opportunities may also be pursued through sabbatical leaves for faculty to enhance their clinical skills. Involvement in private or group practice, consultation, and other personally negotiated arrangements may be used to update or maintain clinical competence. The move toward nurse-managed centers provides opportunities not only for the practice of nursing but also for teaching and research.

ENHANCING COLLEGIAL ROLES

The collegial roles of nursing education and nursing service may be enhanced in several ways. Faculty appointments—adjunct or visiting—represent a mechanism whereby leaders in nursing service may make significant contributions to nursing education. Nursing scholars who hold credentials equal to those required for faculty appointment within the university are recruited and appointed to the faculty. They receive remuneration for their teaching from the university.

Part-time instructors who are engaged in the practice of nursing, usually in the agencies where students are placed, may also be recruited to serve as clinical instructors or preceptors to nursing students. Thus, practicing nurse clinicians are involved in clinical teaching of students. Their role is clear, and their faculty status and salary are determined by the policies of the employing institution. Some health care agencies utilize preceptorship responsibilities for recognition of merit within their own agencies.

EFFECTIVE COLLABORATION

How does one achieve effective collaboration between nursing education and nursing service? No matter which model is used, one must remember that *people* will determine its effectiveness. Collaboration, as used here, means cooperating with an agency with which one is not immediately connected. The relationships among people in the educational institution and the health care agencies are the key determinants of collaboration. Cooperation, effective communication, and compatibility are important ingredients. Styles identifies a hierarchy of elements in collaboration consisting of people, purposes, principles, and structure.[6] People are the base, with purposes and principles determining the structure for building a collaborative endeavor.

Nursing education must have adequate and appropriate resources to

---

[6] Margretta M. Styles, "Reflections on Collaboration and Unification," *Image: The Journal of Nursing Scholarship* 16 (Winter 1984): 21–23.

achieve its goals. Nursing service or practice depends on people who are educated to provide leadership in the health care system. We must make the most of this symbiotic relationship.

In his key concepts for the success of collaboration Walker includes (1) realistic expectations of one another, (2) willingness to accept responsibility for helping each other, and (3) flexibility. Productive collaboration requires mutual respect, trust, and a commitment to the power and strength of a support system in nursing.[7] Nursing must look to nurses for its direction. Ways to promote and structure collaborative relationships must be examined and reviewed continuously. Advisory committees, joint research committees, joint meetings with nursing educators and nursing service representatives, and appropriate contractual arrangements for particular functions are useful.

Most of the models for joint faculty appointments exist within the traditional institutional settings. To promote the idea of unifying nursing education and nursing service and to focus primarily on the hospital setting is shortsighted. Such approaches focus solely on sickness and minimize attention to the increasing need for nursing and health services to both the sick and the well outside of institutions. Forty percent of the 1.7 million practicing registered nurses are currently practicing outside of hospitals. Faculty, therefore, must continue to direct their efforts to innovative and nontraditional practice models in a broad range of settings wherever people are—at home, at work, or in the community. Such opportunities are essential in arranging optimal learning experience to prepare new graduates to seek and carve out new roles in the community, in the broadest sense of the word.

MARKETABILITY OF FACULTY

Do joint faculty appointments make faculty more marketable? According to *Webster's Third New International Dictionary*, something is marketable when "wanted by purchasers." In settings committed to a model requiring faculty to have competence in the clinical practice of nursing, marketability would appear to be a "natural." But what about the marketability of faculty in other settings?

Certainly, faculty are equally as marketable for faculty appointments in colleges and universities that do not embrace the joint faculty appointment concept. The differences occur in how one sets the objectives or goals within the institution for the faculty. Ford and Kitzman believe that marketability of faculty who are qualified for joint appointment is appreciable

---

[7] Duane D. Walker, "Nursing Education and Service: The Payoffs of Partnership," *Nursing & Health Care* 6 (April 1985): 189–191.

in consultation, independent or group practice, joint practice, clinical research projects, or other areas.[8]

PROFESSIONAL ROLE DEVELOPMENT

Do joint faculty appointments enhance or inhibit professional role development? Is the responsibility of faculty for nursing practice an added burden, or is it indeed a functional component of the fully developed professional role?[9] Professional role development is a crucial concern for individual faculty members and their administration. Questions have been raised regarding the extent to which clinical expertise is or is not recognized and rewarded within educational settings. A faculty member whose interests relate directly to clinical nursing should be quite clear about the philosophy of the institution with regard to the faculty role.

Perhaps more questions have been raised here than answered. Economic and social pressures will increase the future demands on nursing and health care. They will continue to increase and become even more complex. I hope that each of us will continue fulfilling nursing's commitment to practice in our diverse ways, but always remembering that nursing, as a learned profession, is both an art and a science.

---

[8] L. C. Ford and H. J. Kitzman, "Organizational Perspectives on Faculty Practice: Issues and Challenges," in *Structure to Outcome*, 13–29.

[9] Joel, "Stepchildren in the Family."

A MODEL OF COLLABORATIVE EDUCATION

PLANNING AND IMPLEMENTING A COLLABORATIVE PROGRAM

GAIL KUHN WEISSMAN, RN, FAAN
Vice-President, Nursing
The Mount Sinai Medical Center
New York, New York

Investigation into creative educational programs has always been a goal for the Nursing Department at Mount Sinai. In late 1979 and early 1980, however, the declining availability of registered nurses precipitated an earnest review of the situation. A driving factor in Mount Sinai's interest in establishing a collaborative education program was its interest in retaining professional registered nurses of the highest calibre.[1]

HISTORICAL PERSPECTIVE

To develop the board of trustees' and administration's understanding of the issues in nurse staffing and how the national picture was affecting

---

These three papers present the experience of the specially designed Mount Sinai Hospital–Pace University Lienhard School of Nursing Bachelor of Science in Nursing Program.

[1] "Strategic Guidelines Addressing Problems of Nurse Recruitment and Retention" (New York: The Mount Sinai Medical Center, Department of Nursing, 1982).

the institution, I recommended that the board of trustees of The Mount Sinai Medical Center establish the Nursing Care Subcommittee of the board's Patient Care Committee. Nursing and hospital administration outlined the complex aspects of the problem, identified the approaches to solving the problem, and set the targets and deadlines to be met. The board committee reviewed management's plans, gave their support to the plans, and made sure that the goals of the plans were achieved.[2]

The institution undertook an extensive study of the evidence of a shortage of registered nurses; the reasons why such a shortage might exist; and the future of professional nursing, including the direction in which the profession will be moving and the reasons for that direction. Reasons found for the decreasing supply of registered nurses had to do with the emotional demands of the job, inconvenient and undesirable working hours, inadequate salaries, insensitivity of hospital management to employees' needs, undesirable locations (that is, in the inner city), and the lack of real educational opportunities.[3]

Members of the board who were on the Nursing Care Committee had been active with the Mount Sinai School of Nursing, which graduated its last class in 1973. Historically, the hospital-based school was a primary source of nurses for the hospital. Therefore, a feasibility study was conducted in 1980–81 to determine whether reopening the Mount Sinai School of Nursing would serve to feed new nurse graduates to the hospital. Because there are now three major types of educational programs, the issue was not only whether to reopen a school, but what type of school should be considered.

Each of the three types of educational programs—diploma, associate, and baccalaureate—was analyzed in terms of its stature within the nursing profession, trends in admissions and graduates, appropriateness for a medical center, cost to establish, and process for obtaining state approval. The completed analysis indicated that reestablishing the Mount Sinai School of Nursing would not produce the desired results.

The second phase of the nursing school feasibility study was conducted to determine if reopening a Mount Sinai School of Nursing as a work-study BSN program for recent diploma and associate degree graduates from regional programs would serve as a primary feeder of new graduates for the hospital. A survey questionnaire was sent to 100 diploma programs accredited by the National League for Nursing and to 71 NLN-accredited associate degree programs in Connecticut, Massachusetts, New Jersey,

---

[2]"Nursing and Patient Care: 1980–1982" (New York: Nursing Care Committee of the Patient Care Committee of The Mount Sinai Medical Center, Board of Trustees, 1982); and "Management Target Dates: Short and Long Term Nursing Staffing Plan, July 1980–December 1985" (New York: The Mount Sinai Medical Center, Department of Nursing, 1985).

[3]W. Feigin, "Registered Nurses: Requirements, Supply and Their Future," paper prepared for The Mount Sinai Medical Center, September 1980.

New York, and Pennsylvania. The response rates were 55 percent from the diploma schools and 58 percent from the associate degree programs.

The data from the survey indicated that reopening the Mount Sinai School of Nursing as a work-study BSN program would not assure The Mount Sinai Hospital a significant number of recent graduates. Recent graduates, although interested in pursuing a BSN, were not likely to relocate to New York City for that purpose. In light of the questionable marketability of the concept, it was therefore considered inadvisable to proceed with reopening of the school, given the costs involved in operating such a program and the difficulties and uncertainties involved in getting New York State approval.

However, the data also indicated that the response might be different from the single diploma graduate with no dependents and for the graduate from a New York City area diploma or associate degree program. The accessibility and availability of a hospital-endorsed work-study arrangement might attract such graduates to The Mount Sinai Hospital for their first position. Such an arrangement could be developed by The Mount Sinai Hospital in conjunction with an existing New York City BSN program.

In May 1983, a Professional Nurse Profile Survey was conducted by the Department of Nursing to provide a data base regarding the professional background of the registered nurses on staff. Data was requested via questionnaire from all 1,312 full-time and part-time professional nurses. The response rate to the survey was 89 percent. Nearly one-third of the sample reported interest in a work-study program at The Mount Sinai Hospital leading to a bachelor's degree. Nearly two-thirds expressed interest in a master's work-study program. Over two-thirds indicated that they would enroll in a degree-granting program in nursing if selected courses were offered at the hospital as an additional academic campus.[4]

COLLABORATIVE PROGRAM

The collaborative Bachelor of Science in Nursing program of The Mount Sinai Hospital and Pace University Lienhard School of Nursing was established in fall 1984. It assists professional registered nurses to further their professional goals by making it possible to earn a baccalaureate degree in nursing at Pace University Lienhard School of Nursing while simultaneously practicing nursing at The Mount Sinai Hospital. This program prepares with the baccalaureate degree professional registered nurses whose initial education was either at the diploma or associate degree level.

---

[4]E. Barrett and R. Wieczorek, "Professional Nurse Profile: Phase I Report" (New York: The Mount Sinai Medical Center, Department of Nursing, March 1984).

Objectives

The students are provided with the same formal program as other Pace students; however, the barriers of time and place that frequently limit participation in higher education are eliminated. The objectives of the collaborative program are the following:

- To enhance the Mount Sinai recruitment and retention program by providing a means for nurses on staff and newly hired nurses to pursue formal education in nursing.
- To enhance the quality of nursing service delivery by promoting an expanded knowledge base for nurses through baccalaureate education.
- To assist nursing service personnel in identifying and meeting their educational needs while pursuing the practice of their profession.
- To promote professional interdependence, collaboration, and accountability in the delivery of health care through a conjoint model for clinicians and academicians.

Program Development

A joint steering committee, consisting of the heads of the Lienhard School of Nursing's programs and nursing administrators from The Mount Sinai Medical Center, was essential in the development and implementation of the program. The involvement of key people from each institution who can facilitate the program in their respective departments—including the dean of the School of Nursing, the vice-president of nursing (or the equivalent), and their top administrative staff—is crucial to the success of such a collaborative program.

Funding of scholarship awards is being sought to give the professional registered nurse the opportunity to complete the program in an abbreviated period of time by taking a semester off from work if desired. Criteria for Mount Sinai scholarships are a grade point average of 3.0 from the School of Nursing and a performance appraisal rating consistent with the institution's Career Pathways Program.[5] Consideration for scholarship awards will be based on employment and current status in the program. Nurses who receive a scholarship will be expected to continue practicing nursing at The Mount Sinai Hospital for a designated period after receiving their degrees.

A letter of understanding is in effect between The Mount Sinai Hospital

---

[5]"Career Pathways: Clinical, Administrative and Education/Research Ladder" (New York: The Mount Sinai Medical Center, Department of Nursing, March 1985).

and Lienhard School of Nursing. In addition to the standard terms of an affiliation agreement, the letter indicates that they are affiliated institutions and may establish joint appointments of individuals to function in the dual capacity of nurse educator for the School of Nursing and nursing service professional (clinician-administrator) for the hospital. The institutions may agree to the exchange of staff and faculty in accordance with the institutions' established standards and policies. The names of individuals who will participate in such an exchange, their credentials, the period of their service, and details of payment or reimbursement, if any, shall be set forth in advance in a mutual agreement, on the recommendation of the joint steering committee. Each institution retains at all times the right to terminate these staff agreements.

The goals of these joint appointments are to:

- Promote advancement of nursing practice and education.
- Provide involvement of faculty in the development and maintenance of standards of nursing practice.
- Advance nursing knowledge through nursing research
- Provide opportunities to exercise the faculty consultant role in clinical practice.

Mount Sinai and Pace will continue to explore creative experimental models for educating both graduate and undergraduate registered nurses in a tertiary care center and will jointly pursue financial support for such endeavors. Both institutions are committed to working in a collaborative effort to provide joint workshops and educational programs for faculty, nursing staff, and members of the professional community.

UNIQUE FEATURES OF THE COLLABORATIVE PROGRAM

RITA REIS WIECZOREK, EdD, RN, FAAN
Assistant Director of Nursing
Clinical Resource Division and Clinical Career Pathway
The Mount Sinai Medical Center
New York, New York

Every successful academic program is composed of unique features which are directed to the marketing of the program to the student population. The particular features of The Mount Sinai Hospital–Pace University Lienhard School of Nursing Collaborative BSN Program have contributed to the program's apparent success.

In the Mount Sinai–Pace program, special attention is focused on the needs of the adult learner. Students in the collaborative program are not in same program as the basic generic baccalaureate students. Nurses are given opportunities in the classroom to apply knowledge and skills learned in the practice setting.

The Mount Sinai Hospital has a Nurse Career Counseling Service available to nurses on all three shifts. Individual or group meetings are made by appointment Monday through Friday. The nurse career counselors are available to offer guidance and assistance to students in the collaborative BSN program in planning professional development directed toward individual nursing career goals and in advancing their formal educational background for nursing practice. The nurse career counselors offer specific services to students of the collaborative program, including:

- Application to the collaborative program—help in filling out the necessary forms for application to Pace University. It is possible to complete the forms at Mount Sinai during a lunch hour or after work.
- Assistance with obtaining transcripts from educational programs, from high school graduation through all types of educational programs.
- Suggestions for writing a personal statement for college or university admission. This is strongly suggested for potential students with weak academic records.
- Suggestions for obtaining letters of reference for college or university admission from individuals who can evaluate a candidate's potential for academic success.
- Educational counseling for the matriculation process.
- Educational counseling for course work and program planning in the collaborative program.

MARKETING THE PROGRAM

Marketing the program was the joint responsibility of the hospital and university. The nurse career counselors implemented a series of orientation programs with Pace faculty and admission officers for the nurses at the hospital. Nurses attending orientation sessions filled out initial interest forms containing demographic data and the necessary information for follow up. The nurse career counselors contacted these individuals and made individual or group appointments for question-and-answer sessions about the new program.

The nurse career counselors developed a brochure that was used internally with nursing staff and as a recruitment tool at job fairs and orientation sessions for newly hired staff members. The nurse career counselors also used the brochure at other professional meetings to familiarize as many people as possible with the new collaborative program.

Presentations were made to trustees, management, and staff groups to inform them about the new program and to gain their support for it. Mount Sinai felt that it was making a real, tangible commitment to facilitate the educational advancement of their nurses. In essence, it was eliminating all the old, standard reasons given by nurses who say they cannot return to school because "it is too inconvenient." The nurse career counselors began to track all potential and actually enrolled students. This was done both as a marketing aid and for follow-up studies.

PROGRAM SCHEDULING AND FEATURES

Every effort was made to provide a flexible work schedule for nurses who enrolled in the Mount Sinai–Pace collaborative program. The vice-president for nursing sent a letter to supervisors expressing support for the program and asking them to consider the educational needs of their staff when planning their unit work schedules. Selected courses are offered on-site at The Mount Sinai Hospital, which has resulted in small classes in familiar surroundings. It also saves the travel time required to attend most traditional programs. Classes in the new program are offered in the late afternoon and early evening hours. The two classes offered each semester at the hospital are given back to back on the same evening for the students' convenience. In addition, some nurses also attend courses offered at Pace University's New York City Campus.

Students in the new collaborative program can avail themselves of Pace University's multiple campuses and university events. If space permits, nurses from other institutions may register for the classes offered at Mount Sinai.

Pace faculty have office space assigned to them in the hospital to facilitate academic counseling and program planning. Thus, Mount Sinai nurses can have an appointment with their professor either before or following classes scheduled at the hospital.

ADMINISTRATIVE FEATURES

The joint steering committee is responsible for the administration of the collaborative program. The chair and meeting place of the committee rotate between the two institutions. The steering committee's activities consist of:

- Approving applications for joint appointees—faculty consultants to Nursing Services and professional nurses to Pace University.
- Requesting annual reports from joint appointees.
- Reviewing the current program and making recommendations for its support and future direction.
- Facilitating course offerings at the Mount Sinai Campus.
- Identifying marketing strategies.
- Developing a research design for the evaluation of the program.

In addition, an advisory committee of alumni, nurses, and consumers has been appointed to support the development of the new program membership.

Tuition reimbursement is a contractual matter at Mount Sinai Hospital in the Department of Nursing. Based on the 1983–86 collective bargaining agreement, nurses who are employed full-time are entitled to tuition aid. Nurses have to have had one year nursing experience and have been matriculated in a degree-granting program to receive this benefit. At Mount Sinai Hospital nurses must apply for tuition aid no later than the second week of a course. Students who successfully complete their courses and document passing grades, receive tuition reimbursement. Thus, nurses need to be able to cover one semester's tuition costs before their benefit assists them with expenses. Pace University was very helpful in setting up a special plan to allow nurses enough time to pay for their tuition, so that nurses could not say that they were unable to return to school because they did not have money. Pace University was willing to help students obtain and make the necessary financial arrangements.

In summary, it is the unique features of the Mount Sinai–Pace collaborative program such as those described here that have made it a success. The support system in the hospital and university setting has been strong, and nurses have responded to the program in a very positive manner. We are hoping that the satisfied students currently attending the collaborative program will market the program to the next group of new students!

COLLABORATIVE BACCALAUREATE EDUCATION FOR RNS RETURNING TO SCHOOL

MARILYN JAFFE-RUIZ, EdD, RN, CS
Chairperson, BS Program
Lienhard School of Nursing
Pace University
New York, New York

In 1962, I heard rumblings about the fact that a BSN was going to be required of all registered nurses. I reacted then with the fear and anger shared by many other nurses who felt as if the rules were being changed midstream. Many nurses thought somehow that it would never mean *them*, a denial that has only allowed them to postpone the inevitable.

The memory of those feelings and frustrations as I embarked on my own return to school is what prompts my commitment to chairing an upper-division baccalaureate program and to the implementation of the collaborative educational experience shared by The Mount Sinai Hospital and Pace University, Lienhard School of Nursing.

Everyone knows how difficult school can be, especially if one is also juggling work and family. The philosophy of the collaborative educational program is very much in keeping with the Pace University motto, *Opportunitas*. Opportunity is provided for the RN working at The Mount Sinai Hospital to return to school at Pace University with a minimum of hassle and a maximum of sensitivity and assistance. For that to happen, administrative commitment is needed from both institutions.

COLLABORATION

Key people are needed from the team representing each institution to operationalize the program. Mount Sinai provided a counselor from their Department of Career Pathways, and Lienhard School of Nursing provided the assistant dean and myself, the chairperson of the BS program, at different times. These people, along with other administrators from both institutions, sat on the steering committee. The Mount Sinai counselor attended and participated in the monthly BS department meetings at Pace. This was a valuable way to bring Mount Sinai to faculty in the department and to place the educational issues of this program in context with the department's offerings.

Continuous dialogue is needed between the key people from each team so that necessary collaborative planning and implementation can take place while enforcing for the RN student that "work is work" and "school is school." Resources from both institutions must be coordinated and the people involved must have their fingers on the pulse of all the activity related to the program while ensuring that confidentiality is maintained. For example, Pace keeps student files containing academic information, and the Department of Career Pathways at Mount Sinai maintains records on those nurses they counsel. However, neither set of files is open to the other institution.

Other departments of the medical center and university must also be involved. At Mount Sinai the library purchased books and put readings on reserve, and the book store made required texts available. Classroom schedulers were extremely helpful and cooperative in providing classroom space. At Pace University, the admissions office, the registrar and the bursar worked with us extensively to facilitate procedures for the students, as did the biology and chemistry departments, which also offered courses on site at Mount Sinai. Students were issued Pace University identification cards at time of registration so that all the facilities of the university, as well as those of the medical center, were available to them.

Students were also offered a policy of prompt tuition remission. Faculty members facilitated this by providing Mount Sinai with grades immediately after the course was over so that checks could be processed without waiting for distribution of official grade reports from the registrar.

It was also crucial to have the support from both institutions for audiovisual materials, printing, transportation money and secretarial support services. Both Pace and Mount Sinai could not have been more generous.

Numerous on-site orientations, open houses, and opportunities for academic advisement were made available throughout the year as well as on-site admissions counseling and registration. Mt. Sinai provided classroom and meeting space as well as an instructor's office. Wine and cheese parties have been hosted for all who have participated in the program or are thinking of enrolling.

The program has been very successful thus far. Thirty students enrolled in the first on-site nursing course in fall 1984. In the spring semester, 15 had enrolled for the on-site nursing course, while the others chose to take courses on the main campus. Only two students dropped out of the program entirely.

RETURNING TO SCHOOL

Students have anxiety and trepidation about returning to school. Clinical courses in particular arouse fears of being a "student nurse" again. Many have unpleasant memories of being degraded and demeaned, with loss of self-esteem. Other disconcerting situations may arise. For example, a woman who was a nursing supervisor when I was in my senior year at Mount Sinai is now a student in my class; she was initially uncomfortable and so was I. Many RN students have a wealth of knowledge and experience—especially since Mount Sinai has excellent staff development and clinical resource programs—but have resisted formal education. This program is an excellent opportunity for them.

There has been some concern about the homogeneity of a work group being in school together. Some students responded to the peer pressure and support in a positive way. Others felt self-conscious and would have preferred greater anonymity. All share the Mount Sinai perspective or vision. On the other hand, all Pace nursing students have the opportunity to register for courses held at Mount Sinai and all the Mount Sinai students have the option of taking the same courses on the Pace campus. Some students have preferred to do this. It is important to keep in mind that only some courses will be offered at Mount Sinai each semester, and students are expected to take only beginning courses at the hospital. It is not intended that the complete program be offered on site.

Some students are reluctant to travel the short distance between the hospital and the university. Fear of the perils of the New York City subway may really be a manifestation of fear of exposure to others outside the familiar institution. A buddy system helps to work out the academic and logistical problems.

Nurses who graduated from diploma schools, worked at the same hospital for many years, and may even live in the neighborhood—frequently in hospital housing—have a certain provincialism. This can be seen in some of the Mount Sinai graduates who graduated prior to 1970 and are now in this program.

By the same token, faculty members who are teaching off campus also experience a sense of disorientation—almost like the awareness during the first home visit of being in someone else's house. The students are a group with a common identity—a family; the faculty member may feel like an outsider. For this reason, only experienced faculty should teach on-site.

Continuation of the collaborative baccalaurate degree program is essential. As the proposal to require the baccalaureate degree for RNs becomes a reality, more opportunities must be made to facilitate the return to school for registered nurses.

THE ROLE OF NURSING ADMINISTRATION IN FACILITATING NURSING RESEARCH

RENA M. MURTHA, MA, RN
Associate Director for Nursing
Clinical Center
National Institutes of Health
Bethesda, Maryland

The integration of nursing research into practice settings has evolved gradually in the last several years. Until recently, most nurse executives have not been faced with the notion of personal or organizational support for nursing research. Nursing research has been something that took place in academe and was conducted by those in the profession endowed with time, motivation, and grants to conduct studies of importance to the profession.

DEVELOPMENT OF RESEARCH IN PRACTICE

Historically, nurse researchers have been predominately faculty members who either devoted themselves solely to the conduct of research or who, in order to survive, had to conduct research and publish. Little has been reported in the annals of nursing research about the development and encouragement of research conducted in practice settings. Nevertheless, nurse administrators are now being encouraged and in some cases are encouraging others to develop the notion of conducting research into practice, education, and administrative issues in the workplace. Slowly, a small cadre of clinical researchers have moved into practice settings, first as consultants, then as part-time or joint appointees, and finally as full-time employed nurse researchers on the staffs of medical centers, home health agencies and long-term care facilities.

In the 1970s, as an outgrowth of support for nursing research from the Division of Nursing of the U. S. Public Health Service, the Council of Nurse Research Facilitators was developed to bring together researchers and others who were encouraging and supporting research in all spheres of the profession. The council is a vehicle for new ideas, encouragement, collaboration, and networking in support of nursing research.

Typical of nursing, the development of research in practice settings is fraught with conflict. In this era of cost containment and realignment many nurse executives have identified the need for solid data to defend their practice methods, staffing patterns, organizational designs, productivity, and a myriad of other practices that are under attack. Moreover, nurses need to disavow ourselves of the notion that the only workplace for nurses is the hospital. Nursing research needs to be developed in a variety of arenas, therefore, if we are to conduct meaningful, replicative research. Nursing is caught in the dilemma of an increasing need to justify all it stands for with resources to build substantive arguments becoming scarcer than ever.

The American Organization of Nurse Executives, in their series on Nurse Executive Management Strategies, issued a document entitled *Integration of Nursing Research into the Practice Setting*, which urged that nurse executives "view the environment's economic constraints as an incentive to the integration of nursing research into the practice setting, instead of a prohibiting factor." In support of this position,

> Nurse executives that maintain practice-based nursing research programs report program costs to be justified in view of departmental savings associated with productive and efficient methods of nursing care delivery validated by research. Program costs are further justified as nurse executives identify cost effective methods of nursing care delivery that facilitate institutional adherence to DRG limits on patient lengths of stay.[1]

OPTIONS FOR COLLABORATION

The key to success in the development of the programs currently used by nurse executives to integrate nursing research into the practice setting is collaboration and the encouragement of colleagueship. Gone are the days of the nurse administrator and nursing school dean operating *in*

---

[1] American Organization of Nurse Executives, *Integration of Nursing Research into Practice Settings* (Chicago, Ill.: American Hospital Association, 1985).

vacuo. The "*town-gown*" dichotomy within nursing must disappear if nursing research is to flourish.

Consultation

Many nurse administrators of patient care facilities initially develop cooperative agreements between their nursing services and schools of nursing to provide consultation to nursing service in developing research questions and to serve as mentors to staff in various aspects of research design and methodology. Usually the faculty member enters the practice setting through the nursing education department. The first project is generally a survey course in nursing research for interested staff. The nurse researcher frequently is employed as a consultant to the nursing administrator in the area of design and methodology.

Research Committee

Many institutions utilize the researcher only as consultant on a sporadic basis. The second step is to employ the nurse researcher on a consultative basis to provide direction to a committee, usually made up of head nurses and clinical specialists, created to formally develop nursing research questions at an organizational level. The consultant is seldom able to conduct her own research but is mainly employed to advise institutional employees who have developed their own studies. The nurse researcher in this case may be one of many individuals from academe who may have an interest in research but who is not employed as a full-time nurse researcher. Access to patient populations for nurses interested in doing research is usually determined by the committee members, medical staff, and clinical interest of staff represented on the research committee or staff accessing the committee for mentoring.

Development of a research committee is an evolutionary and in some institutions revolutionary step. Committees have emerged from journal clubs, faculty practice groups, and special project groups, and finally develop into officially sanctioned committees. Since most organizations have few staff members who have conducted their own research, the consultant's first responsibility is to provide staff development in the areas of problem identification; the research process, including the library search; research methodology; and data collection and analysis. Over time, committee members begin to assume a mentorship role as well as an educational one for new staff interested in conducting studies with more seasoned investigators. Access to the human subjects review committee in most institutions must be facilitated by the nursing administrator and nursing research consultant.

Joint Appointment

Some nursing administrators have entered into agreements with graduate schools of nursing to provide for a joint appointment of a full- or part-time doctorally prepared nurse researcher. In an era of declining revenue, both facilities tend to profit by such an agreement. The school of nursing is able to participate in funded projects in research and gains access to staff and clinical facilities to conduct research. The patient care facility has the services of a fully prepared researcher to develop studies that benefit both organizations while establishing nursing research as a positive force in the organization. Staff development and continuing education programs are also made available to staff at no additional cost to the organization.

Full-Time Nurse Researcher

Finally about 65 practice institutions at this time have established a full-time position for a nurse researcher. These nurse researchers are members of the department of nursing and in some cases hold the combined title of director of research and education. They often have adjunct appointments at one or more universities so that they maintain collegial relationships with teaching institutions. They serve as grant writer, principal investigator, educator, mentor, spokesperson, and advocate for nursing researcher as well as consultant to or chair of a nursing research committee where one has been established.

In institutions where nursing research has been encouraged and developed, educational programs are organized for staff and colleagues and the results of studies are published to share the results of the research with the profession.

ROLE OF NURSING ADMINISTRATOR

The nursing administrator has an educational as well as administrative role in this process of developing a research program. Few physicians and administrators view nursing as a sophisticated and scientifically based profession able to conduct its own research at a sufficiently scientific level to warrant their approbation. The nursing administrator must be knowledgeable in concepts of nursing research so that she can prepare administrators, physicians, department heads, and staff to accept nursing research as a needed and important aspect of the organization.

The issue of resource allocation is critical in the development of nursing research endeavors in clinical practice settings. Nursing administrators and researchers must be clear as to what is to be researched to make maximum use of data and resources and they must be knowledgeable about grant writing and funding sources. They must also be informed about previously reported studies that may be further developed and are defensible to avoid duplication of effort. They must collaborate on studies with other organizations interested in similar information—hence, the need for colleagueship. It is more important than ever to the future of nursing research that we stick to researching the critical issues that improve our efficiency and cost-effectiveness rather than conducting studies on topics that are "nice to know about." A nursing administrator can amortize the cost of conducting research and employing a nurse researcher by developing research questions and data that improve the organization of the delivery of nursing care.

NURSING RESEARCH AT THE CLINICAL CENTER

The evolution of nursing research at the Clinical Center of the National Institutes of Health (NIH) is an example of the development of a cost-effective research program over time. The mission of NIH is to provide support for biomedical research. The Clinical Center was opened in 1953 to provide a site for the consolidation of the intramural programs of the various institutes. Initially, the administrative philosophy stated that only those employed to conduct biomedical research would be permitted to conduct research at the facility. Hence, those professionals employed to "support" research—that is, those employed in social work, laboratories, radiology, nursing, blood bank, and so forth—were not permitted to conduct their own research.

In 1978, the administration agreed to support the concept that to enhance biomedical research it was important for research to be conducted in all aspects of the institution. That year the first nurse researcher was recruited, a nursing research review committee was established, and staff were encouraged to develop clinical questions.

From 1978 to 1981, the nursing research committee developed bylaws and standards of research. The committee began to work with the MD, PhD investigators to develop nursing research questions that frequently paralleled biomedical research. Some nurses mistook the process of gathering data for biomedical research for nursing research and required assistance in understanding the definition of nursing research. In the early days of nursing research at the Clinical Center, the staff was offered considerable education and mentoring in the maze of the research process.

Nursing research at the Clinical Center has evolved from a committee of interested, committed neophytes to what it is today. It has followed the path of recruiting one person alone as nurse researcher, without support staff. In 1985, a full-time doctorally prepared nurse researcher carries the title of director of research and education and senior nurse scientist. The committee's bylaws have evolved into a formal, approved definition of nursing research, a specific role for chair and members, consultation by the senior nurse scientist, and a formal reporting mechanism and review that complies with the federal guidelines for research. All nursing research protocols involving patient populations must be defended by the nurse principal investigator before an institute institutional review board (as must those of all scientists) as well as meet the approval of the nursing research committee. Endorsement must be obtained from the associate director for nursing and the director of the Clinical Center. All nursing research is catalogued and receives a protocol number. The researcher protocol must contain an approved informed consent document and submit to periodic review.

Staff nurse job descriptions have been rewritten to include expectations of the development and participation in nursing research. Head nurses are required to provide staff with time for library searches, data gathering, and committee support as the work of the unit permits. Studies are encouraged and supported in all aspects of nursing, clinical practice, education, and administration. The initial orientation for all professional nurses includes a module on the research process. A staff development program taught by the director of research and education for nursing is available on methods and concepts of nursing research. In addition, all institute institutional review boards have a member of the Clinical Center nursing staff as a permanent member.

In 1985, two intergovernmental personnel agreements were specifically earmarked for nursing research. This provides an opportunity for two additional doctorally prepared nurse researchers to spend from six months to two years at the NIH Clinical Center to conduct research and to serve as mentors to staff and students. Twelve graduate programs are now affiliated with the Nursing Department of the Clinical Center, four at the doctoral level. This provides students with the opportunity to develop research questions utilizing the staff and patient populations available at the Clinical Center facility.

The director of research and education has developed a nursing research review panel so that proposed studies and those in process may be overseen by recognized members of the nursing research community. Finally, the Nursing Department is in the process of developing the potential for an international exchange program in nursing research that will parallel the international scientist exchange program conducted through the Fogarty International Center at NIH. This will provide nurse researchers from other countries with the opportunity to work with us in developing nursing research that benefits nursing internationally.

In 1984, the Nursing Department had some 21 protocols at varying stages of development and published over 70 articles in refereed journals.

The department sponsors an annual nursing research symposium, which is another vehicle for the dissemination of the nursing research being conducted at the Clinical Center. In fiscal year 1986, for the first time in history, NIH and the Clinical Center Nursing Department will sponsor the first consensus conference in nursing developed on an issue that has been investigated in depth by the profession.

Nursing has a distinct advantage at the Clinical Center. Nursing is at the heart of the success of biomedical research, and nursing is respected and encouraged at NIH. However, nursing research is still an infant. We have come a long way but we still have miles to go. Our goal for the future is to develop targeted research based on quality assurance studies and issues important to the future of the profession and NIH.

CONCLUSION

As a profession, nursing continues to repeat our history. Development and facilitation of nursing research is a crucial issue in this decade. Nursing administrators are being called upon daily to prove and defend all their recommendations and decisions. The solution is sound, scientifically based research. This can be the arena in which the profession unites around education, practice, and administration. I believe strongly in the notions of collaboration and collegiality. We are nothing alone. We need to share ideas, research, and people. Without the ability to do nursing research, someone else will do it for us, and the outcome may not be to our liking. It certainly has not been in the past. There are no guarantees it will change. For the future, there can be no question that without research conducted by nurses, for nurses, in the best interest of nursing, there will be no future.

RURAL NURSING AND THE MALDISTRIBUTION OF NURSES

SANDRA STUART-SIDDAL, MS, RN
Director, Rural Nurse Placement Center
California State University, Chico

By definition, *rural* means "country," a term that distinguishes rural areas from the cities or towns where populations are massed together. Statistically, a rural community has a population of 2,500 or less. A more realistic definition in terms of the communities that rural nurses serve would be between 500 and 1,000 people. *Rural* designates a sparsely populated area where the economy is based on industries such as agriculture or logging. These industries usually take up large blocks of land. People and buildings are not clustered together in a rural community; there is no real center to the population.

Most rural townsfolk live a Spartan existence, free of luxuries and marked by simplicity and frugality. Rural days are slower, the social life is markedly restricted, there is far more isolation and greater distances between neighbors. People are conservative, concerned with the basics of life. The work ethic is still very important. The notions of big government and welfare are unacceptable. Rural people are strong, individualistic, independent, and opinionated.

People in rural areas still leave their doors unlocked or leave keys in the ignitions of trucks or cars. Business can still be done on a word-of-mouth basis. If a stranger comes into town, townsfolk view him or her with curiosity. If the stranger is willing to work, play, and live by the community

117

rules, he or she can stay. If the stranger wants to change anything, he or she is ostracized.

Outdoor recreation, canning, and gardening, are the leisure activities in these communities. These are places where everyone knows everyone else's business, gossip is still an accepted form of communication, the work of a person is still valued, and "trust" is still a strong value.

PROBLEMS OF RURAL HEALTH CARE

An element of self-care and folk medicine is practiced in most rural environments, both by need and by choice. The lack of health care providers in those areas makes it necessary for rural folk to be able to take care of most of their own health needs. By choice, they tend to prefer non-traditional approaches to medicine and thus practice folk medicine, use herbs, and favor natural living and eating.

The independent, provincial rural person will not travel any great distance to seek out health care, even in what most urban folks would consider an emergency situation. The rural folk will just "tough it out." That same independent attitude prevents a lot of people from getting a variety of preventive health services, such as blood pressure screening, physicals, well baby care, immunization, or family planning, that are aimed at taking care of the body, maintaining health, or getting well.

An additional problem is the lack of adequate resources for referral. For example, mental health services are virtually nonexistent in rural areas. Anyone in a crisis gets only temporary and nonspecific psychiatric intervention from the closest acute-care hospital or clinic. Long-term care is next to impossible to find. Most other health referral services, social services, and therapy services are lacking in rural areas as well.

Health care can also be a financial burden. Most rural people have no health insurance or group coverage through employment. Many rural folk are self-employed or are employed at low wages, and make just enough to survive on. Most rural residents are supported by such industries as mining, farming, ranching, logging, forestry, and tourism. Historically, and at this time in particular, these industries do not provide high-paying jobs. Needless to say, limited personal financial resources or insurance policies limit access to health care.

PATIENT CHARACTERISTICS

There are specific characteristics that define the type of patient who needs nursing care in a rural area. Although the characteristics of these people may overlap with those of any sample of patients in any hospital, they have some unique qualities to be found only in rural areas. Thus, the rural nurse has to adapt to dealing with these specific characteristics, that no other group needs to deal with.

First, as noted, rural residents frequently will not seek medical attention until a condition is well into pathology. This is based on some relatively simple factors and attitudes, some of which have already been mentioned:

- Lack of money to get treatment.
- Lack of awareness of any medical assistance for which they might qualify.
- Pride in independence and desire to avoid using federal or state aid.
- Belief that "If I tough it out, it will go away."

Second, most rural folks will not pursue any follow-up care. The nursing staff has to do everything on the patients' first visit, for the chances of them coming back once the crisis is over for patient education or preventive education and reevaluation of the condition, is slight. Therefore, the nurse has to take an aggressive approach to the patient in the rural setting different than that used in the urban or suburban settings.

Finally, nurses in small towns usually know their patients personally or know of them. This also forces a different approach to the immediate and ongoing care of patients in rural areas.

These characteristics dictate certain other approaches on the part of the rural nurse. Because most rural town residents are poor, nurses and physicians must take into consideration the economics of the region and the patient's financial status in making any care plans that require medical supplies, prescriptions, or long-term care. Moreover, even though nurses need to appreciate and respect the desires of the rural population for more nontraditional medical approaches than we may be used to, educating the populace about traditional approaches is still necessary. Ignorance is deadly and may cost someone his or her life. If people rely too much on home remedies or have too great a fear of being treated in a clinic or hospital, they may not seek help from a traditional health care person in an emergency, even if that person is next door.

RURAL NURSES AND THEIR WORKING ENVIRONMENT

Given the problems inherent in rural living and the characteristics of the rural population, the role of the rural nurse should be easier to understand. Among the characteristics of the rural nurse are the following:

- Applies the nurse practice acts to their maximum extent and depth.

- Is more diversified than most urban or suburban nurses in his or her practice and job role.

- Is a *generalist* who has to be current in all the nursing specialties and more. When left in charge of the hospital, she or he is the one to make the decisions for all the medical-surgical, obstetrics, pediatrics, intensive care, critical care, emergency room, psychiatric and geriatric patients. With no code team to call or dietary division with which to plan special meals, the rural nurse assesses, plans, carries out, and evaluates all the nursing care for the patient and activates the protocols when the physician is not accessible. As several rural directors of nursing service have noted, the rural nurse must be very flexible. Within hours she or he may be called upon to help with a delivery in obstetrics or a cardiac arrest in the emergency room, to interpret an arrhythmia in the critical care unit, to console a family, or to assist with the care of auto accident victims. The nurse may also have to spread salt on icy walks, plunge toilets, or mop up the delivery room. There is no real preparation for this type of work. One also must be able to tolerate slow days when nothing is happening, but think and work hard and fast when everything seems to be going on at once.

- Generally is a paramedic or emergency medical technician, has a coronary care certificate, and is prepared to handle just about any emergency or set of circumstances thrown at him or her.

- Gets more involved with the people. She or he gets involved personally and emotionally with most of the patients who walk through the door. In a rural community, nurses see many of their patients repeatedly and cannot escape that relationship as one can hiding in the maze of a large city or town.

- Has a closer working relationship with the physicians and more contact with the hospital administration.

- Has to teach preventive health techniques and theory as much as possible to patients to counterbalance the rural "tough-it-out" attitude and practice of folk medicine and self-care.

- Is assertive.

- Is aggressive when necessary.

- Is autonomous in his or her role.

- Is independent in decision making.

- Carries more than one job role within the facility. One nurse may be the utilization review person, the emergency medical technician, and the inservice director.

Rural nurses must also contend with a fluctuating house census, which affects the number of days they can work per pay period. Directors of nursing service may have to hire part-time people to maintain coverage. It is nearly impossible to entice RNs to a rural community and hospital when the offer is part-time, no benefits!

Rural areas throughout the country have always experienced a shortage of nurses. Most rural facilities are understaffed, and there are no nursing pools to draw from if current staff members are ill, on vacation, or on leave. The staff who remain must take on heavier loads, assume more responsibility, and put in longer hours. In one hospital in Northern California, two RNs staffed a hospital for a two-month period by themselves, by splitting the day into two shifts, just to keep the hospital doors open! Access to nursing registries from the nearest city area is also poor because the limited financial resources of the small rural facilities prevents them from paying the exorbitant registry fees. Moreover, the distances involved are just too great for most registries to be able to get nurses to agree to go to rural areas.

Because the distances to the urban centers are often so great and access to physicians limited, the majority of emergency patients that come to a rural facility receive initial lifesaving measures and intervention from nurses. If possible, they are flown to an urban center later when they are stable enough. Rural nurses have to act alone, utilizing standard procedures and protocols—and they do a magnificent job!

Finally, since sophisticated follow-up and referral service is nearly impossible in a rural town, the nursing staff also has to be responsible for discharge planning that is realistically oriented to the situation and the independent attitude of the typical residents.

MALDISTRIBUTION OF NURSES

The maldistribution of health care professionals is one of the major problems of America's health care delivery system. Rural communities in particular suffer from a lack of physicians and nurses. The Rural Clinical Nurse Placement Center (RCNP), located at California State University, Chico, helps to address this problem by introducing nursing students to the professional and personal experiences of living and working in rural communities through six- to eight-week experiences that allow students to better consider employment in rural areas. RCNP participants are given a thorough introduction to the rural experience that frequently results in participants' returning to practice in rural communities.

Although the maldistribution of physicians has been the subject of numerous studies and corrective programs, the maldistribution of nurses is just beginning to be addressed. Professional factors usually cited for the lack of nurses in rural communities include lower salaries, fewer opportunities for advancement, reduced access to continuing education, less exposure to unusual patient cases, less contact with professional peers, and fewer nursing specialities. Personal deterrents to living in rural communities are isolation from cultural and recreational activities, fewer employment opportunities for mates, housing shortages, and extreme weather conditions. Although these factors do exist, the RCNP believes they do not by themselves explain the maldistribution of nurses, and they can be balanced or outweighed by other factors unique to rural communities. For the nurse in his or her professional role, these factors include the opportunities to develop a greater number and variety of skills; to accept more on-the-job responsibility and independence; and to relate to physicians, nurses, and patients on a more personal level. For the nurse as a member of the community, these factors include a more relaxed pace of life, a sense of community, and environmental beauty and purity.

The RCNP addresses four specific underlying causes of the maldistribution of nurses.

The Lack of Awareness of the Rural Experience. Many nurses were raised or attended nursing schools in urban or suburban communities. As a result, nurses are generally unfamiliar with the rural experience and with the demands and rewards of rural nursing. They simply do not consider rural nursing as a career option. The RCNP increases awareness about the rural experience through its on-campus recruitment efforts, presentations at conferences and professional meetings, a 30-minute color film and a 20-minute slide-tape presentation about the program, and various publications and brochures. The growing number of inquiries about the program indicates that these consciousness-raising efforts are producing results.

The Urban Bias of Nursing Education. Most nursing programs tend to acculturate their students, however subtly, to the role of the urban nurse. Most nursing schools are located in urban or suburban communities, as are most of the hospitals, clinics, and public health departments in which nursing students are trained. The standard for job comparison soon becomes the urban experience: the sophistication of specialized care and equipment, the professional credentials of co-workers, the potential for professional advancement, and so on. To the uninformed, rural nursing pales by comparison. But rural nursing is a speciality in its own right. It entails a different kind of sophistication—a jack-of-all-trades independence; different credentials for co-workers—capability, dependability, and personality; and different potentials for advancement—community respect, peer admiration, and personal satisfaction. By exposing nursing students to these standards, the RCNP adds a much-needed perspective and balance to the urban bias.

The High Drop-Out Rate of Nurses.   Reasons given by nurses for leaving the profession include lack of opportunity to learn new skills, poor worker communication, high patient-nurse ratios, less patient contact and more paperwork, and lack of respect from physicians. These complaints are rarely heard among rural nurses. The nature of rural nursing is such that learning new skills is not only possible but necessary; worker co-operation is essential; lower patient-nurse ratios are the rule; patient contact is assured; and respect from physicians is more freely given. Rural nursing may be the ideal alternative for urban nurses who have left or may leave nursing for these reasons. By returning these nurses to the rural labor force, the RCNP increases not only the number of nurses in rural areas but the number of nurses in the state as well.

The Difficulty of Relocation.   Unless nurses have contacts in rural communities, they may never be exposed to a catalyst for the move to a specific rural community. Rural health facilities seldom have the resources they need to recruit for nursing positions. Staff members may not be available for recruitment work; the facility frequently needs physicians, laboratory technicians, or X-ray technicians as badly as it needs nurses; and the money for advertising may not last until the position can be filled. The RCNP experience and the professional and personal relationships it involves increases the ease with which participants—and their friends—can relocate in rural communities. Familiarity with specific rural communities, health care facilities, and residents is a decided advantage in choosing a work setting, finding housing, and establishing oneself in a new community. The RCNP can be the catalyst that turns the inclination toward rural nursing into a reality.

CONCLUSION

Thus, the RCNP is addressing the maldistribution of nurses by raising awareness about the rural experience, by adding a needed perspective to the urban bias of nursing education, by offering unemployed nurses an alternative kind of nursing practice, and by increasing the ease with which nurses can relocate in rural communities. The premise is that these activities will attract nurses to rural areas, and the evidence thus far indicates that this is the case. Although the RCNP is making an impact on the nursing shortage in rural areas, the need is still great for these unique, highly versatile professionals—rural nurses.

EDUCATIONAL AND CLINICAL PERSPECTIVES IN ALCOHOLISM

MADELINE A. NAEGLE, PhD, RN
Associate Professor
Lienhard School of Nursing
Pace University
Pleasantville, New York

Recent developments in scientific, social, and professional spheres bring new perspectives to understanding and addressing the phenomenon of alcoholism as it relates to nursing. These developments represent departures from past thinking and shape educational objectives for health care professionals as well as for those involved in their basic preparation. These important trends include changes in scientific and attitudinal designations of the disease of alcoholism; clearly defined approaches to treatment, including designated nursing roles; action by professional groups to identify and assist practitioners suffering from the disease; and social action directed toward prevention and containment of the problem.

CHANGING VIEWS OF ALCOHOLISM

One important change is the shift from the perspective that alcoholism is a bad habit, a personal weakness, or merely a symptom of deeper unresolved conflicts. There is an increasing acceptance of the correspondence between patterns of alcoholism and the epidemiologic model of disease. Detection and treatment now focus on the phenomenon as a chronic, progressive, psychophysiological process, which, while not curable, can be arrested through intervention and the assumption of a drug-free life style.

The extent of the problem, which makes it an important public health issue, is more openly acknowledged. Alcoholism afflicts as many as ten million people and ranks among the five most prominent diseases responsible for morbidity and mortality rates in the United States. The nature of its social consequences has led to speculation that the problems of each individual alcoholic affects at least four other people—family members, co-workers, or friends. The prevalence of the problem and the extent to which it goes untreated ensure that all practitioners of nursing, regardless of practice setting or specialty area of concentration, will encounter the alcoholic or members of his or her family.

Important new trends in research on alcohol use and its effects have strongly influenced the size, nature, and scope of the knowledge base about patterns of alcohol consumption. Although previous studies focused largely on individuals with the disease, recent investigations explore the relationships between alcoholism and constitutional factors, such as endogenous opiates; specific risks to health associated with alcoholism, including early death and myocardial infarction; and alcohol use and preventable conditions, such as fetal alcohol effects and fetal alcohol syndrome.[1] In addition, studies are now designed to focus on the needs of specific groups such as women, children of alcoholics, and ethnic minorities.

Biological studies are yielding data that increase the understanding of phenomena associated with alcoholism, such as tolerance—the cellular adaptation to increasing amounts of the drug—and withdrawal—the reversal of adaptive cellular and tissue changes. Such studies supply evidence of the far-reaching effects of alcohol on the central nervous system and major body organs.

This understanding of alcoholism and its associated complex psychological and physiological processes has broad educational implications. Teaching must include the implications of alcohol's use for health as well as the identifiable consequences that occur in a disease state following long-term abuse. Curriculum content in basic and continuing nursing education programs must reflect the extent and comprehensive nature of the disease and include the wide scope of nursing interventions appropriate to its manifestations in acute and chronic phases and to primary,

---

[1] G. A. Olson, P. D. Olson, and A. J. Kastin, "Endogenous Opiates: 1983," *Peptides* 5 (1984):975–992; S. Deutscher, H. E. Rockette, and V. Krishnaswami, "Evaluation of Habitual Excessive Alcohol Consumption on Myocardial Infarction Risk in Coronary Disease Patients," *American Heart Journal* 108 (1984):988—995; *Medical World News* (New York) November 12, 1984; and E. M. Ouilette, "Fetal Alcohol Syndrome," in *Developmental Handicaps: Prevention and Treatment II* (Silver Spring, Md.: American Association of University Affiliated Programs, 1984).

secondary, and tertiary prevention. Nursing functions can be described for all of these levels and for varying degrees of professional skill. The nursing knowledge base for alcoholism in the areas of health maintenance, assessment, nursing care, and evaluation should approach that for other major diseases.

APPROACHES TO TREATMENT

A far greater amount of information is now available to support the likelihood of positive treatment outcomes for alcoholism. Primary impediments to curriculum change and the development of clinical expertise in this area have been the negative attitudes of health professionals about the alcoholic as a patient responsive to medical and nursing care and pessimism about the possibilities of recovery.[2] Although research findings that correlate treatment modalities with successful outcomes are still limited in number, the visibility of recovering alcoholics in public life, professional groups, and the business community has done much to change stereotypical attitudes about the disease and its responsiveness to treatment.

Change in attitude has been identified as an important curriculum goal if educators expect health care professionals to care effectively for the alcoholic client.[3] Experiential teaching methodologies should be part of medical, nursing, and other curricula, including such techniques as panel presentations by health professionals who are recovering from alcoholism, attendance at an Alcoholics Anonymous or Al-Anon meeting, and educational sessions with children of alcoholics.

As nurses incorporate new knowledge about alcoholism into existing structures, the implications for the application of such knowledge and the development of nursing roles become more clear. At the generalist level, curriculum content on alcoholism can be integrated into existing structures, so that students are able to derive specific nursing approaches to this illness for broader nursing principles. Examples of this include the utilization of assessment and interviewing skills, utilization of community resources in care, and the application of family theory to the dysfunctional alcoholic family. Generalist practitioners need to learn to manage the health care of alcoholic clients and their families by implementing the nursing process and incorporating community and interdisciplinary re-

[2] R. Cornish and M. Miller, "Attitudes of Registered Nurses Toward the Alcoholic," *Journal of Psychosocial Nursing and Mental Health Services* (December 1976): 98–109; and E. Hanna, "Attitudes Toward Problem Drinkers," *Journal of Studies on Alcohol* 39 (1978):98–109.

[3] J. Hostetler, *Alcohol and Drug Abuse Teaching Methodologies Guide for Medical Faculty* (Rockville, Md.: U.S. Department of Health and Human Services, 1982).

sources into care in an approach similar to that used with other diseases. These possibilities, however, are not sufficiently reflected in current educational practices.

PROFESSIONAL ACTIVITY

The nursing profession is according new attention to the educational preparation and role functions of the nurse in the specialty area of substance abuse. Such attention includes active exploration of such questions as, What are nurses contributing to research on this and related phenomena? How does nursing intervention differ from approaches utilized by social workers and alcoholism counselors? What credentials are important and necessary for specialization in this work? At present, members of specialty nursing organizations with a primary focus on clinical issues in drug and alcoholism nursing and the American Nurses' Association (ANA), are collaborating on the development of standards of practice for substance abuse nursing. The description and delineation of the nursing role in this specialty is essential to the establishment of nurses' credibility as providers of care for the alcoholic patient.

Another important trend in professional activity has been the initiation of formal action by state and national nurses' associations to address the incidence of alcoholism among professional nurses. Recognition that professional nursing practice can be impaired by excessive use of and addiction to alcohol or other drugs was formally recognized in a resolution passed by the ANA House of Delegates in 1982. The resolution identified clear ethical direction in the activities it proposed for the organization, including education and peer assistance.[4] Since then, activities in the forms of peer-assistance programs, legislation to provide alternatives to licensure revocation, and seminars and workshops on impaired practice have been widespread.

Responsibility for regulating high standards of nursing practice is inherent in professional education and the concept of professional accountability. Nurses need to be educated about the personal risks of addictive illness, the detection and management of impaired practice, and the ethical aspects of nurses' rights in the employment setting. The average nurse knows little about such important considerations as the conditions that support the development and continuation of impaired practice or collective bargaining issues related to employee benefits, such as sick leave and coverage for treatment of substance abuse illness.

---

[4] M. A. Naegle, ed., *Addictions and Psychological Dysfunctions in Nursing: The Profession's Response to the Problem* (Kansas City, Mo.: American Nurses' Association, 1984).

SOCIAL ACTION

A number of social developments have enhanced the educational climate for both the layperson and the professional. The social response to the consequences of alcoholism increases the importance of acknowledging aspects of the problem in practice and education. The level of public awareness of the dangers of alcohol use and abuse is gradually rising, and group action has brought about legal and social changes. Examples include efforts to raise the legal drinking age, stricter enforcement of detection and discipline of drivers who are intoxicated, and lobbying to restrict liquor advertising in the media. Groups such as Mothers Against Drunk Driving (MADD) and Students Against Drunk Driving (SADD) have gained visibility in their efforts to educate others about the social and economic as well as personal consequences of alcoholism.

These informal social controls and legal sanctions change attitudes and the drinking climate. Such a focus on alcoholism as a social problem, however, does not necessarily increase the understanding of it as a disease; and such a designation is essential to obtaining funding for research and to bringing about change in the formal education of health professionals. Nevertheless, looking at the situation optimistically, public health problems that become public causes often receive acknowledgement.

CURRICULUM OBJECTIVES

These developments, as well as new knowledge about alcoholism, provide both an impetus for change in educational approaches and the content to implement that change. Specific implications for learning must be derived by each professional discipline, and levels of nursing education must necessarily identify appropriate objectives about alcoholism. However, curriculum goals identified by Gallant for health professionals can be modified to provide objectives appropriate to the generalist nurse practitioner.[5] They would include the following:

1. Assessment of personal attitudes about drinking and the alcoholic client. Of particular importance is the ability to be empathic to the individual whose self-destructive behavior is socially deviant and damaging to health.

2. Identification of the major types of psychodynamic mechanisms and psychological symptoms that are predisposing factors or consequences of substance abuse.

---

[5] D. Gallant, *Alcohol and Drug Abuse Curriculum Guide for Psychiatry Faculty*, Health Professions Education Curriculum Resource Series (Rockville, Md.: U.S. Department of Health and Human Services, 1982).

3. Identification of the disease process in all its phases and utilization of interventions that are phase related.
4. Definition of essential elements of the therapeutic nurse-client relationship.
5. Identification of appropriate treatment techniques and implementation of strategies to involve the client in treatment, such as detoxification, rehabilitation, or health maintenance.
6. Implementation of primary, secondary, and tertiary prevention strategies in institutional and community settings.

Curricula designed to meet these objectives, whether in basic nursing programs or continuing education, will provide the nurse with a knowledge base about alcoholism and appropriate nursing interventions comparable to nursing knowledge about other diseases. The application of such knowledge will necessarily be a function of educational preparation and functional role within various settings. This basic preparation will also provide opportunities to further delineate nursing roles with clients who have substance abuse problems. As nurses recognize the disease and its predisposition and consequences as an appropriate area for nursing research, further opportunities for nursing involvement will develop. The study and treatment of alcoholism is still a new area. Its parameters are unclear, but the relevance and importance of nurses as health care providers in the field are not. The challenge to nurses is to define the nature and scope of the nursing role and nursing activities related to alcoholism.

BIBLIOGRAPHY

Burkhalter, P. *Nursing Care of the Alcoholic and Drug Abuser.* New York: McGraw-Hill Book Co., 1975.

——— "Alcoholism, Drug Abuse and Addiction: A Study of Nursing Education." *Journal of Nursing Education* 14 (April 1975): 30–36.

Chodoroff, B. "Student Nurses: Relationship of Personal Characteristics, Attitudes Toward Alcoholism and Achievement. *Quarterly Journal of Studies of Alcohol* 30 (1979): 657–664.

Estes, N., and E. Heineman, eds. *Alcoholism: Development, Consequences and Interventions.* St. Louis, Mo.: C. V. Mosby Co., 1982.

Hanna, E. "Attitudes Toward Problem Drinkers." *Journal of Studies on Alcohol,* 39 (1978): 98–109.

Hasselblad, J. *Alcohol Abuse Curriculum Guide for the Nurse Practitioner.* Rockville, Md.: National Clearinghouse for Alcohol Information, 1984.

Mendelson, J., and V. Mello. *The Diagnosis and Treatment of Alcoholism.* New York: McGraw-Hill Book Co., 1979.

INTERNATIONAL NURSING EXCHANGE: THE UNITED STATES AND CHINA

KATHLEEN M. DIRSCHEL, PhD, RN
Dean, Graduate School of Nursing
Vice-Chancellor, University of Massachusetts at Worcester

Perhaps the farthest reaching possibility for international nursing exchange lies with the United States and China. Geographically, China is 12,000 miles from the United States—a 12-hour time difference—as far away as it is possible to be on this planet. Our governments operate on opposite principles: autocratic versus democratic. Our official family and social policies are different: Two children (recently increased from one) are allowed per family in China, and having more children results in a pay deduction for each one. Children are encouraged in the United States, and each new child *increases* the tax deduction. Dress and personal liberties are markedly different in the two countries, as is the concept of "freedom."

One of China's major political tenets concerning health care delivery is that "medicine should serve the workers, peasants, and soldiers." Yet China's health delivery service has had to contend with the extensive health needs of a vast country with a poor, unevenly distributed, predominantly rural population. Indeed, the population is immense; one billion people are scattered over 3½ million square miles, with 80 percent of them in the rural areas. Technology is far behind Western and Eastern nations alike. Travel is slow, as is communication between provinces.

Moreover, more than 200 million of China's people are of school age.

This school-age population, equal to the entire population of the United States, suffers from extremely limited teaching resources. In many towns even blackboards and erasers are nonexistent. However, China's limitations in technology, equipment, and library resources are significantly counterbalanced by an all-consuming thirst for knowledge and the driving motivation to learn. This enthusiasm for learning, which has burgeoned after the Cultural Revolution, is a force that will help propel the Chinese into the twentieth century in terms of knowledge and technology. It was this force that reached across time and oceans and eventually led to a nursing exchange program with Seton Hall University.

ORIGINS OF THE NURSING EXCHANGE PROGRAM

In 1980, China approached several colleges and universities in the United States, including Seton Hall University, with a proposition for educational and cultural exchanges. The schools that were selected had a history of Chinese study or some other connection with mainland China. A delegation from the State of New Jersey sponsored by Seton Hall was put together in the spring of 1980. I was included both as an administrative representative of Seton Hall and also as the official escort to Jean Byrne, the wife of the then governor of New Jersey, Brendan Byrne, who otherwise would have been the only woman.

Once the delegation arrived in China, my background as a nurse educator became known, and I visited hospitals and schools of nursing in several cities. They were enlightening visits. Like their counterparts in the United States, nurses in China are struggling with low pay, poor public image, and relationships with doctors. But there were many differences as well. Nursing students are "chosen" by the government and have little chance to change their life's direction. Working conditions and learning conditions are poor. The environments are dull and dark, not very sanitary or conducive to learning. Library resources are virtually nonexistent because most written materials were destroyed during the Cultural Revolution. Teaching is by formal lectures in which faculty members read from textbooks. Students dutifully listen and take notes but do not question or enter into dialogue.

What is lacking in give and take, however, was more than made up for in motivation to learn. In all my years as an educator, I have never experienced the degree of eagerness to learn that was exhibited by the Chinese students. A society that combined Western technology and science with Eastern tenacity and motivation would be the highest form of society. Exchange programs, such as the one established with Seton Hall, can be the stimulus for combining the best of diverse cultures, while reinforcing what is similar.

131

The exchange program between Seton Hall and several schools in China took shape after several visits to the People's Republic of China to discuss terms and conditions. At present, it has several facets. The Chinese select the discipline—usually medical/surgical, obstetrics, and pediatric nursing—about nine months prior to the exchange visit. The faculty members are selected and agreed to by lengthy international correspondence, as are the content areas, details of scheduling, and so forth.

Nursing faculty from Seton Hall (usually two at a time) teach in their discipline in a hospital in the city of Hangzhou. They may teach as many as 200 doctors and nurses in two sections of 100 each. The students—nursing students, nursing faculty, nursing staff, and physicians—are selected and brought together by the health minister and the nursing leaders of the province. Most of them work in the hospitals of the province, but some come from outside. The teaching components take about three weeks. Translators are provided. Classroom, seminar, and clinical experiences are part of the teaching. There are also official meetings, banquets, and visits. The faculty members' last week in China is spent touring in the Hangzhou area, Peking, and Shanghai. The costs of the touring, as well as all living expenses in China, are borne by the Chinese provincial governments and schools.

Seton Hall faculty have also taught in the neighboring province of Wuhan. Most recently they have served as consultants to the Second Medical College of Shanghai, where the first BSN program is slated to begin. The exchange program has also sent a large teaching and touring group. Seventeen nurses from Seton Hall and cooperating institutions participated. Based in Shanghai, these nurses taught more than 900 nurses and doctors during their two-week stay.

Also as a result of the exchange program, Seton Hall College of Nursing currently is sponsoring a student from Shanghai who is studying here for the MPA. In the future, we hope to be able to sponsor a nursing student. The major obstacle has been their limited command of English.

The Seton Hall exchange program with China provides a framework for consideration of the role of nursing in the world health community and the impact of exchanging ideas between diverse cultures.

ROLE OF NURSING IN CHINA

The nations of the world, especially third world nations, have a shortage of health personnel, particularly nurses and doctors. China is a prime example of this. This shortage is producing a serious gap in the delivery of services to certain segments of the population, especially the peasants and working class. Despite their limited numbers, nurses are still the most numerous single group of health personnel and often form the backbone of family health services.

In China, nurses are essentially subservient to physicians and to the patient's family. Nurses primarily take directions from physicians. Their practice generally consists of comfort and custodial measures. A large part of their work is learning about and administering herbal medicines. Nurses in China also face a dilemma about how to manage and administer patient care, because of the large role family members play in this area. During the Cultural Revolution, there were even fewer nurses and doctors. Accordingly, families were strongly encouraged by the health care institutions to administer patient care. Families thus became dominant in making health care decisions with regard to the patient.

The dominance of the family and the power of the physician still are to some degree major barriers to the development of the nursing role in China. Efforts are now being made to renegotiate the balance of power, so that the nurse and the doctor form a professional "team," with family and patient membership. To this end, American nurses have been able to provide role models for guidance, consultation, and stimulation of ideas to promote a larger voice for nurses in patient care protocols.

Since the teaching and consulting exchange program also involves physicians and health care administrators, the program stimulates awareness of change in the nurses' role at a multidisciplinary level. The nurses' role as presented and discussed contains the following components:

- *Hands-on caregiver.* Again, U.S. nurses must bear in mind that in China the family still plays a large role in this area and that the hands-on care is less complex than that in the "high-tech" Western nations.

- *Teacher of home care and self-care* to the patient and the family. Although this role is well developed in the United States, it is only just beginning in countries such as China. Teaching is not yet considered a significant part of health care.

- *Coordinator/manager of patient care.* Nurses in China function in traditional head nurse and staff nurse managerial roles. At present, patient assignment is made by the head nurse after degree of acuity is determined by the physician. It would be desirable to realign these determinations so that there is more nursing input. Concepts of accountability, responsibility, interpersonal relations, physician-nurse relations, personnel and organizational management, and patient assessment and triage are covered.

In addition, Western concepts and treatment are presented in the exchange program's teaching. These ideas are combined with Eastern beliefs in energy diversion through acupuncture, herbal medicine, moxibustion, and the use of time to heal to create a unique, encompassing approach to care.

A unique role for nursing is emerging in China. The suppression of nursing's voice and the limited opportunity for scholarly learning reduced the quality of patient care considerably during the Cultural Revolution. Yet the need for prepared personnel, who in many instances are the only caregivers, has served as a catalyst for nursing education. In China, as more and more patients are using hospital facilities, nurses are being seen more and more as direct caregivers and as teachers of patient care and have a greater voice in determining their own role in relation to physicians and families. Chinese nurses are beginning to be recognized as a powerful and useful force in the health care delivery system. In order to develop their role, Western concepts of nursing care are being gradually introduced. Change will be slow, but what will emerge is a nurse with the unique resources of Eastern caring, timelessness, and herbal and acupuncture treatments, combined with Western assessment, scientific inquiry, and pharmaceutical miracles. Both East and West have much to learn about this new universal nurse.

IMPACT OF DIFFERENT CULTURES

The Western nurse in a third world country such as China is faced with drastic differences in living styles, resources, and attitudes and practices in health care. As noted, there is forceful propaganda aimed at maintaining family size of only one or two children per family. Although people in the United States are also reducing the numbers of children per family, it is ostensibly their choice and not imposed by the government. Poverty is widespread in China, but there is a deserved pride that the Chinese are clothed and reasonably well fed—no small task with a population of more than one billion. Dress throughout the country is similar. Health care practices that we take for granted—such as brushing teeth, using a flush toilet system, or separating sick babies from well babies in the hospital—are generally unknown. Delivery of health care is based on payment by the government, also the source of salaries.

The stark differences between East and West are reflected in nursing and health care. There is relatively little high-technology care; there is little follow-up home care; there is extensive use of herbs. There are no such concepts as nursing diagnosis, primary nursing, or nursing theory. Our thrust for cost-efficient care is not a concern.

As already described, resources for treatment are limited or nonexistent. In China I saw blankets that were more patch than blanket. Healing occurs more by time than by active treatment. It makes little difference how long patients stay in hospitals. Teaching is by formal lecture, sometimes read. Students do not question. They are, however, glued to every word of the teacher's. Everyone studies English.

The Western nurse who enters this culture comes from a very different environment for learning and practice. Time is of the essence in Western culture. We are expected to treat the patients quickly with every resource at hand and then empty the hospital bed. Resources are plentiful and all but totally disposable. Although this is beginning to change somewhat, it is a pervasive attitude in Western health care.

The Chinese have little knowledge of Western nursing care and a great deal of pride in their own country and their own ways. But they also have a strong desire to learn about Western ideas and to meld them with those of the East as well as a hope that things will not change too quickly.

Taking these cultural differences into consideration, several implications emerge for a nursing exchange with a country such as China. English must be included among the subjects taught, so that study in the United States is more feasible for Chinese nurses and so that they can read American books and journals. Because there is still little distinction between what is medicine and what is nursing, careful teaching of the similarities and differences between the two professions should also be addressed. Physicians are still the primary teachers of nurses, so the preparation of teachers is of paramount importance.

Understanding and respect for cultural differences must be a part of any teaching or clinical experience. Integration of both cultures in the delivery of health care is the key to success for Western nurses working in China. In that country, the best therapeutic results are obtained by a mingling of the traditional Chinese and Western medicine. In the nursing arena this implies several strategies for the emerging profession, such as the affirmation of respect for the profession among Chinese nurses through learning about nursing theory, nursing process, nursing diagnosis, and nursing organizations and exploring the physician-nurse relationship.

RECIPROCAL BENEFITS OF AN EXCHANGE OF IDEAS

It is important to emphasize that the benefits of an exchange program are reciprocal. The value of any exchange program is *not* to "Americanize" the other country, but rather to share ideas and knowledge. Significant benefits reaped from the China exchange have included the collection of data for intercultural research on such variables as expression of pain and locus of control; the opportunity to provide significant consultative services to China as they move into baccalaureate nursing education; and the opportunity to teach physicians as well as nurses about nursing care, health care, and health care delivery. These mixed classes are the beginnings of dialogue between the professions.

One of the most obvious benefits of an exchange program is the cross-fertilization of ideas and a deeper respect for both cultural similarities and differences. Individuals who participate in the managing or the teaching and learning aspects of any exchange program will be personally and professionally enriched. In addition to the personal knowledge gained, an important by-product is the sharing of this knowledge with others. Through the presentation of papers, through written articles and mono-graphs, disseminating the views of other cultures and describing their interrelationships with ours create understanding between peoples that may lead to more respectful relationships between countries. Drawing people together through the understanding of cultural beliefs and the intermingling of ideas and technologies will ultimately help all nations to achieve better coping skills for the twenty-first century.

quality and ethics

THE FUTURE OF NURSING IN THE ACUTE-CARE SETTING: IMPACT ON NURSING CURRICULA

KATHERINE W. VESTAL, PhD, RN
Associate Executive Director
Hermann Hospital
Houston, Texas

Nursing in the acute-care setting is currently undergoing such rapid change that it is difficult to try to predict future scenarios. Changes in finance, care resources, and technology have all affected the acute-care facilities and moved nursing into a dominant position in the hospital business.

The twenty-first century is only 15 years away. We are currently making decisions, both in delivery of services and in the preparation of providers, that will determine the scope of acute health care in the year 2000. Issues such as access to services, quality of services, technology, regulation, physician practice, hospital systems, and new health care ventures are all currently undergoing changes. Issues of productivity, capital funding, coalitions, and the medically underinsured client are equally important.

These issues and others will have profound effects on the type of nurse needed in acute-care settings. Nursing education and nursing service must collaborate carefully to produce a nurse who can function effectively in the new health care arena.

DOMINANT TRENDS

Although many trends are currently receiving attention, those of the increase in aging population, health care cost containment, competition in health care, and increasingly complex technology will have a direct impact on the educational preparation of a nurse.

The aging population has received considerable attention with the phenomenon of the "graying of America". It is predicted that by the year 2000, 65 million people will be over the age of 65. Life expectancy continues to lengthen, and as people live longer they are more likely to have increasing health problems. Thus, their need for care in acute-care facilities will rise, and the disproportionately high demand on services will cause a significant increase in resource consumption. Nurses will need a strong background in gerontological nursing as well as new methods of care for the elderly in order to meet this demand.

The current focus on economical health care is bound to continue. As resources get tighter, the need for acceptable quality services delivered by responsible professionals will heighten. Nurses will need to be educated about cost-benefit issues and the economics of care delivery. This education, begun in generic programs, will be emphasized in the work setting on a continuing basis once the nurses enter practice.

Another phenomena that is already affecting acute-care hospitals is the surge of competition in health care. This competition has heightened, requiring hospitals to carefully examine the services they offer. Services must be of the type and cost that will be utilized by consumers, or hospitals will have to find alternative ways to finance the services that are underutilized or not cost-effective. Hospitals are expected to continue to be the focus of health care well into the twenty-first century, so the business side of these services must be considered.

Competition has also raised many questions about the "business" of acute-care facilities. Will hospitals offer services for the sick, for the healthy, or for both? What will be the obligation of the hospital to maintain people at the highest quality of life? The many new health care delivery systems—such as health maintenance organizations, preferred provider organizations, and independent practitioner associations—are altering the health services delivery picture to the point where most acute-care institutions are seriously considering the future nature of their businesses. Competition in health care is reflective of the free enterprise system, focusing on supply and demand and reasonable quality products at affordable prices.

The fourth major trend that will affect nursing service education is the rapid escalation of technology. Technology is changing the face of patient care with improved monitoring and measurement devices and innumerable new methods of moving information. Information technology, or informatics, has thrust acute-care nurses into the role of data processors as they constantly integrate physiological, financial, and environmental data to coordinate and deliver patient services. The use of computers has moved to the forefront as a skill needed by nurses.

Thus, developments in the current era of health care have focused attention on the need for change and development of alternative systems for delivering health care. As a direct result of the prospective payment system, acute-care settings have had to make a critical assessment of their strengths, weaknesses, and future directions. It appears that in the future, patients in hospitals will be more acutely ill, will require services that coordinate and integrate with home and community facilities, and will demand these services to be delivered in the most efficient and productive way possible. The nurse, as the primary care provider in acute-care facilities, has an opportunity to guide the course of hospitalization and to ensure that care is of an acceptable quality. This will require a nurse who is prepared to function in the four basic areas of acute nursing care—clinical, administration, education, and research. The nursing curricula must address these focuses of practice with current information on the needs in those settings.

NURSING CLINICAL PRACTICE

Expectations of the professional nurse in clinical practice continue to increase. Cost constraints require that nurses function in a variety of roles and skills, and these skills must be defined in terms of competencies. The acuity of the conditions of patient population in acute-care settings is increasing, thus demanding higher levels of skill to maintain high-quality care. This high-quality care has communication as its basis, including the ability to successfully communicate with peers, supervisors, patients, families, and other health care providers.

Nursing students are being exposed to acute-care systems that are in a state of flux, during a time when the students are seeking a stable environment in which to learn. Graduate students attempt to intercede at higher levels in order to meet their learning goals. There is no question that opportunities for learning in hospitals are enhanced by the growing sophistication of care strategies and technology, but at the same time, the uncertainties present in the delivery systems challenge the ability of both students and faculty to accomplish learning tasks.

It is ironic that the basic tenets of nursing that have been taught for so long, such as admission assessments, patient-nurse relationships, patient and family teaching, and discharge planning, are now becoming the critical basis for efficient care delivery and provide a perfect opportunity for nursing education and service to share expertise. Curricula must address these basic issues as well as expose students to the newer realities of clinical care such as organ transplantation, noninvasive procedures, new diagnostic modalities, and other sophisticated treatments.

NURSING MANAGEMENT AND ADMINISTRATION

The current and projected economically constrained environment of health care has increased the pressure in service settings for sophisticated nurse managers and administrators. Currently, nursing preparation has varying degrees of managerial content, mostly directed at preparing middle managers.

This preparation may be correct for the graduate nursing student who is seeking a focus in administration. It is increasingly apparent, however, that the undergraduate curricula must also address managerial content to meet the needs of the new nurse. The staff nurse is expected to understand and function within the business arena of nursing as well as the clinical arena. The new staff nurse is finding increasing emphasis on measuring the quality of care, costs, and productivity as well as creating a professional environment for practice. In addition, the new staff nurse needs a basis for good communication, appreciation for the political aspects of the organization, and a sense of the financial implications of patient care services. Pressure for integrated interdisciplinary care is increasing, and new nurses must know how to be team members as well as leaders.

The managerial and administrative aspects of the nurse's role will continue to increase, as the acute health care systems engage in competitive services in a cost-constrained environment. Nurses should begin to deal with these issues as students, rather than being surprised by the harsh realities as they begin to practice.

NURSING EDUCATION

The patient education function of the nurse in acute-care settings is increasing rapidly with the pressure to shorten hospital lengths of stay. More teaching must be accomplished in a shorter period of time, so that patients can meet their care needs in the home environment. In addition, there is a need to teach colleagues and other students new information as it becomes available.

There is a constant need in acute-care settings for teaching all disciplines at various levels, as well as for orientation and updates on new modalities and technologies. In addition, experience has shown that continuing education in the work setting is a major tool in retaining nurses.

Thus, nurses in acute-care settings are finding that they have a teaching role in all facets of health care delivery. They need curriculum support for these programs and practicum experiences with patients and families. Teaching nurses to teach is a constant need in curricula, now and in the future. In addition, universities and hospitals should evaluate their programs to see if they are duplicating offerings, and consolidate resources to ensure high-quality, cost-effective courses.

NURSING RESEARCH

Nursing research is an often-neglected area of nursing in acute-care settings. Particularly as institutions face cost constraints, resources for research tend to decrease, and the hospital is underutilized as a scientific laboratory. Clearly, through nursing research, many of the needed solutions for changes in practice can be determined and new practice methodologies validated. At no time has the need been greater for well-conducted quantitative and qualitative studies of nursing practice in acute-care settings.

Graduate students and faculty will need to work with acute-care nurses to identify and investigate practice problems. Sources of funding must be identified, and collaborative projects between education and service should be developed. Nursing students must be encouraged to apply research findings to enhance patient care and nursing practice.

CONCLUSION

The future of acute-care settings is predictable only from the standpoint of change. There are many variables that will force these systems to find new methods of delivering patient services. Nurses will have a major role in determining the nature of these changes and in implementing new methods of practice. These times need new ideas and new solutions—resources frequently possessed by students.

Nursing curricula must foster inquisitive minds and challenge them to improve nursing practice. The destiny of nursing can be managed by nurses only if the opportunities are seized and acted on. A sense of optimism about the continued development of the acute-care nursing role can be instilled in students by faculty who see these opportunities. It is an exciting time for nurses in acute-care settings. Let's not let it pass us by.

THE CURRICULUM OF THE FUTURE: ADAPTING TO CHANGING DEMANDS IN COMMUNITY HEALTH

LILLIAN M. McCREIGHT, MPH, RN
Assistant Commissioner for Professional Services
State Director of Public Health Nursing
South Carolina Department of Health and Environmental Control
Columbia, South Carolina

Think of current trends in health care delivery, and a number of acronyms leap to mind: DRGs, PPOs, HMOs. One gets a mental picture of new entities in our neighborhoods—surgical centers, emergency care centers, the "doc in the box." We read of ever-expanding technologies of organ transplants, artificial organs, lithotripters, CAT scans, and machines that monitor and sustain every body function—prior to birth, during illness, and past the ever more cloudy point when death occurs. We hear that the increasing number of physicians is having—and will have—a great impact on health care delivery; and there are both optimistic and pessimistic descriptions of those effects.

In the community, these health care trends must be viewed in the context of social and demographic factors: an aging population; a persistent, stubborn infant mortality rate; an openess to variations in sexual behavior; poverty (including hard-core poverty, multigenerational poverty, the newly unemployed poor, and poor single-parent families); and the dilemmas of balancing fiscal soundness and compassionate social responsibility.

The immediate and continuing effect of these health care trends and social factors on community health nursing is the need and demand for more home care. The South Carolina health department, which employs proximately 1,000 public health nurses, saw a growth rate in its nursing staff of 12.6 percent in 1984 and a growth in home care services of 30 percent—and this in a time of fiscal conservatism and budget constraint!

The population receiving home care is growing in variety as well as numbers. In addition to traditional home care patients—the chronically ill, the injured with long-term recovery and rehabilitation needs, and the terminally ill who choose to remain at home—new population groups are confronting home care services. These include the products of early hospital discharges—the acutely ill, who are completing at home what a short time ago would have been an inpatient stay, bringing demands for intensive nursing care and technological miracles with them. Early discharge also affects postpartum patients and their newborn infants; and the trend toward deinstitutionalization of psychiatric care brings a new set of vulnerable people into home settings. "Home care" thus takes on a kaleidoscope of forms and descriptions.

OPPORTUNITIES

Home care is not the only new—or renewed—challenge facing community health nursing. Although much time and effort is devoted to "sick care," community health nursing is still emphasizing prevention in public health. Much of our attention is focused on early detection and prevention of chronic disease, including advocating under the rubric of health promotion the broad changes in life-style that affect later vulnerability to debilitating disease processes.

Whole new horizons open up for community health nursing as we consider the health impact of toxins in the environment and attempt to control the disposal of hazardous materials while developing sensitive measures and systems for monitoring human responses to exposure. Opportunities on this public health frontier for nurses with keen assessment and epidemiological skills are exciting and boundless.

The opportunity to be a public health pioneer in communicable disease also beckons for public health nurses. We are in the forefront of solving the puzzle of acquired immune deficiency syndrome (AIDS) as it creeps into populations other than those first identified as high-risk groups, and the terror of a disease with no known cure escalates. The complexities of other sexually transmitted diseases also present new challenges for public health nurses who serve as primary clinicians in attempts to break the cycle of transmission and reinfection.

Although *The Nation's Health* tells us that tuberculosis is declining, South Carolina continues to have about 500 new cases per year. Public health nurses manage the prevention, case finding, teaching, supervised intermittent therapy, and interpretation to an alarmed community that each case represents.

Epidemiology is not confined to chronic and communicable disease. The same principles, applied by public health nurses in the planning process, are keys to making a difference in infant mortality. Preconceptual intervention programs, risk scoring, and special intervention for prevention of low birth weight, assessment and triage of high-risk pregnancy, and high-risk infant tracking are all based on linking problem analysis to outcomes. These activities, carried out by public health nurses, are making a demonstrable impact on mortality and morbidity in the first year of life.

EDUCATIONAL PREPARATION

Community health nurses are serving as direct care providers, program supervisors and managers, discharge planners, clinicians, evaluators, and administrators. What are we expecting of educational programs to prepare them for these multiple and complex roles?

In the preparation of the public health staff nurse—the backbone of health service delivery in the community—we are looking to baccalaureate programs to prepare *enough* nurses for entry positions. This will allow agencies to redirect resources currently invested in teaching basic principles of public health and basic supervision to nurses whose educational programs lacked this content, but who still comprise the majority of the applicant pool.

Public health employers expect that baccalaureate graduates will come to the job well grounded in essential content and skills needed for practice in any setting: physical assessment, physiology of aging and other aspects of gerontology, growth and development from conception through the life cycle, common pathology, pharmacology, nutrition, psychology, cultural diversity, infection control, basic supervision and management—the list goes on and on. In addition, we expect a firm foundation in public health science: epidemiology, biostatistics, community assessment and organization, home visiting, identification of high-risk populations, program planning and evaluation, public policymaking, and political processes. We are looking for a beginning practitioner who is able to think through situations she has not experienced.

The public health specialist—the product of graduate education—should have built on this foundation to achieve in-depth mastery of the content areas described, plus beginning research skills and broader administrative capabilities.

At all levels of education, we expect to have interwoven inextricably with clinical content the development of interpersonal skills—skills as team players, supervisors, interdisciplinary collaborators, change agents, and teachers of adult learners. Some of this content can be taught didactically and demonstrated clinically—provided the clinical settings practice what is being taught. Some must be role modeled by faculty and clinical preceptors to come alive and be integrated into the student's practice.

This is a tall order, a demanding one, but the practice setting and the needs of the population are what write that order. In public health practice we see ourselves as partners in the educational process, not as critics, aloof and distant. The responsibility is overwhelming, but we offer shoulders—as well as minds, energy, and commitment—to share it.

THE CHANGING HEALTH CARE DELIVERY SYSTEM: THE LONG-TERM CARE PERSPECTIVE

MELANIE P. COX, MS, RN
Corporate Director of Nursing Services
Meridian Healthcare
Towson, Maryland

In the past, long-term care has been the stepchild of the health care system. Its future status may be that of favorite child, for long-term care is the most rapidly growing component of health care in the United States. Most of nursing continues to view long-term care as the stepchild who must be recognized but whose worth or value is questioned. If nursing does not change its attitude, we are going to miss one of the biggest opportunities we have had in years to move nursing forward.

WHAT IS LONG-TERM CARE?

What is long-term care and why is it going to become so important? For the purpose of this paper, long-term care concerns the resident or client who, because of physical and/or mental condition, is unable to cope with tasks of daily living without assistance for an extended period of time. Critical to long-term care is the assumption of responsibility for working in a collaborative way with the individual to assure the provision of the items and services needed to achieve and maintain maximum freedom of activity. The long-term care system should facilitate the arrangement of a variety of formal and informal services to assist the person and the family to achieve and maintain optimal well-being.[1]

Long-term care encompasses a wide range of services both within and outside of the institutional structure. These services include health maintenance, rehabilitation, illness care, personal care, housekeeping, and various levels of assistance with activities of daily living. These services may exist in the organizational structure of a nursing home, a chronic hospital, respite care, hospice, day care, a counseling or support program, or a retirement community—and this list is expanding rapidly.

Simply put, long-term care represents a continuum of care dealing with quality of life for residents and families. The long-term care population encompasses people of all ages and should not be thought of as including only the elderly. Recent estimates suggest that over nine million Americans suffer from severe functional impairments, and this number is expected to grow dramatically during the next 25 years.[2] Reasons for this growth include: (1) the growing number of ill neonates who are surviving with sequelae requiring long-term intervention, (2) an increase in trauma victims who are surviving the trauma but are left with deficits in self-care, (3) a growing number of individuals with terminal illnesses, and (4) the "graying" of America. The elderly constitute the country's most rapidly expanding age group, with most of the increase among those age 85 and older. Of those age 65 and older, only 5 percent utilize nursing home care. In the group referred to as the frail elderly—those 85 and older—many of whom have complex health care needs, 20 percent will utilize nursing home care.[3]

At present, approximately 100,000 nurses work in long-term care. Growth projections estimate the creation of more than 6,000 additional jobs per year.[4] We are repeatedly reminded of reduced census in hospitals, resulting in layoffs for all levels of staff. The job opportunities are going to be in long-term care and home health. Nursing comprises 80 percent of the health professional roles in long-term care.[5] If we do not act now, the challenge will be to maintain that share of the job market. Medicine is

[1] Mildred O. Hogstel, *Management of Personnel in Long-Term Care* (Bowie, Md.: Robert J. Brady Co., 1983), 74–75.

[2] Laura Reif and L. Estes Carroll, "Long-Term Care: New Opportunities for Professional Nursing," in *Nursing in the 1980's: Crisis, Opportunities, Challenges*, ed. Linda H. Aiken (Philadelphia: J. B. Lippincott, 1982), 147–177.

[3] *Facts in Brief on Long Term Health Care* (Washington, D.C.: American Health Care Association, 1984), 11–12.

[4] "Nursing Personnel," *Report to the President and the Congress on the Status of Health Personnel in the United States*, Vol. I, Part C (Washington, D.C.: U.S. Department of Health and Human Services, Division of Nursing, August 1984), C-1-33.

[5] Reif and Carroll, "Long-Term Care," 147–177.

already identifying employment potentials in long-term care, as job opportunities for physicians in hospitals and private practice are reduced.

The response to this challenge begins with the educational system and expands to the profession as a whole in terms of the need for recognition of long-term care's status. Perhaps some of the denigration of long-term care results from hostility toward those we feel impotent to help. And this impotence in long-term care stems from inadequate knowledge, largely a result of the lack of research.

Long-term care nursing is not acute-care nursing practiced in a long-term care setting. The Long-Term Care Committee of the National League for Nursing has been working to identify skills and competencies for long-term care nursing. In a recent article, Brower lists skills and competencies needed for different levels of academic preparation.[6] High on the list, of course, is assessment skills. Variations from the normative state that occur with aging must be an integral component of physical assessment. Assessment skills must also include functional status, mental status, decision-making skills, stress factors, and family structure. Decision-making skills are critical for nurses in long-term care because they receive little backup from physicians. The resident or client depends on nursing's assessment when more intervention than nursing can provide is indicated. Nurses must also become better at identifying options for care and obtaining them. Nurses must develop a working knowledge of payment structures and how these payment mechanisms affect options for care.

NURSING OPPORTUNITIES IN LONG-TERM CARE

Alzheimer's disease may be the fourth leading cause of death in the United States today, and by the year 2020 it will be our leading cause of death. Individuals who reach age 85 have a 30 percent chance of developing Alzheimer's disease.[7] The behavior, problems, and needs of Alzheimer's victims are varied and complex. Nursing needs to do much research in these areas to determine assessments and intervention strategies if we are going to meet these needs.

Nurses also need to understand options in the services available to residents or clients and their families. Day care is a perfect area for nurses to function in, not only as practitioners, but also as entrepreneurs. Whereas owning a nursing home today is difficult for any independent individual, with multifacility enterprises making up 75 percent of the industry, primarily to achieve economies of scale, some of the smaller service options,

---

[6] H. Terri Brower, "Knowledge Competencies in Gerontological Nursing," in *Overcoming the Bias of Ageism in Long-Term Care* (New York: National League for Nursing, 1985), 55–82.

[7] *Alzheimer's Disease: Report of the Secretary's Task Force on Alzheimer's Disease* (Washington, D.C.: U.S. Department of Health and Human Services, September 1984).

such as day care, require little up-front capital and have low fixed costs. Plus, the reimbursement structure is already in existence.

Another area for entrepreneurial development is health maintenance in retirement centers or senior citizen housing. A geriatric nurse practitioner could develop a proposal to market his or her services to a developer of retirement complexes, showing how these services could make the retirement complexes more competitive. Some states now require limited hours of health supervision for retirement centers.

These examples show how nursing can meet the needs of consumers while helping to establish nursing in the business world. Medical schools give courses in how to run one's own business. Does nursing?

There is also a growing need for counseling and support programs for caregivers. The stress of caregivers is being manifested in an increase in abuse of the elderly. The 85-year-old resident of a day care center may have a primary caregiver who is 65 or older. Role reversal is taking place simultaneously with a critical adaptation in the caregiver's own life. Neither life nor nursing education has prepared caregivers for the impact of these stresses. Here again is a need that must be met and could be met perfectly by nursing. If it is not, other disciplines will fill the gap.

Ethics and value clarification are important areas for all students and practitioners. All of us will age and will die. Identifying our values about aging and death can be facilitated with clinical rotations in long-term care if the experience is approached with an open mind. Most elderly people have suffered, have coped, and have learned to deal with life through living itself. Faculty members who have enthusiasm for long-term care nursing can help students gain experientially rather than seeing long-term care as an unchallenging clinical rotation where only basic skills can be learned. Faculty are pivotal in establishing this positive tone.

RESOURCE MANAGEMENT

It is news to none of us that health care today is business—a very big business representing a substantial portion of the gross national product. For years nurses have tried to ignore this fact, almost embarrassed by it. Prospective payment may have forced us to finally become more business oriented, but we still have a way to go.

Stevens recently addressed resource management, saying we should prepare nurses to be resource directed rather than goal directed.[8] One type of resource is, of course, financial. It is important to understand the revenue resource in nursing homes. Approximately 3 percent of nursing home revenues come from Medicare and other third-party payers. Fifty-

---

[8] Barbara J. Stevens, "Tackling a Changing Society Head On," *Nursing & Health Care* 6 (January 1985): 27–30.

two percent comes from state Medicaid systems. That leaves 45 percent of revenues coming from private payments.[9] This revenue base differs greatly from that of acute care and home care. Not only are there revenue constraints created by the states (the 1985 increase in Medicaid for many states was less than 3 percent), but it is difficult to roll over increased costs into the private payment market and remain competitive in terms of market share. Certainly, if 45 percent of hospital bills were paid directly by the public, the hospital picture would be totally different today. It is going to take creative, competent nurse managers in long-term care to come up with proposals that will increase quality of care within the constraints of financial resources.

Another resource is people. All nurses in long-term care are managers to differing degrees based on position, but all levels need basic management skills. The decision-making skills that accompany the nursing process are the same skills that are involved in problem-solving in the manager role. Communication techniques that are effective in the therapeutic relationship between nurse and resident are the same communication skills used by an effective manager. Many nurses resist making those connections, however. They see the roles of clinician and manager as unrelated. These managerial skills need to be presented as more universal, regardless of the nurse's role when she or he utilizes them.

Given current resources, nurses in long-term care will continue in the foreseeable future to have this dual role. This affects preparation for directors of nursing. The director of nursing must have a strong clinical identification, for he or she may be the major clinical resource. Many of us are looking for geriatric nurse practitioners with management skills and experience to serve as directors of nursing in nursing homes. How many master's programs in nursing administration include components of long-term care? Creativity and innovativeness must exist in the top nursing position of any organization. If changes are going to occur at lower levels, upgrading the skills of this key position is crucial.

Corporate nursing management must also be addressed. This is a new phenomenon, but certainly part of the future of nursing management, regardless of the care system. We are just beginning to identify the skills needed as the job develops, but the power in organizations is in the corporate structure, so nursing most assuredly must be at the corporate level.

THE FUTURE OF LONG-TERM CARE

In summary, the growth in health care is going to be in long-term care and home care. Long-term care has residents and families with complex

---

[9] *Facts in Brief on Long-Term Health Care*, 13–19.

needs who require high-quality nursing care at all levels to adequately meet these needs. The structure of the long-term care system requires nurses to be managers as well as clinicians. As the clinical role is complex, so is the management role. The structure of the system is changing, and nurse managers must change with it to better represent nursing within the organizational structure. Educational programs must respond enthusiastically to these needs and help us develop enthusiastic nurses who can see the future and take advantage of the opportunities. Favored-child status for long-term care is going to be much more fun than that of stepchild!

TEACHING ETHICS IN THE NURSING CURRICULUM

MINERVA I. APPLEGATE, EdD, RN
Professor, University of South Florida
College of Nursing
Tampa, Florida

As nurse educators, we have a responsibility to prepare nurses for the real world of nursing practice. How do we prepare nurses to make decisions when the decisions that they are confronted with have ethical overtones, or when nurses find themselves in situations demanding ethical decision making? Nurses are being faced with unprecedented choices as a result of technological advances and new knowledge gained from the sciences. Life is prolonged with life-support systems and new treatments and therapeutic measures. Infants with congenital anomalies now have life prolonged, and questions of the quality of life are presented to the decision maker in such situations. Patients are being exposed to increasingly more invasive procedures as a result of technological advances.

Increasing government regulation has led to greater awareness on the part of the health care consumer. Health care providers are protesting as society imposes external measures to foster the accountability of health care providers for the services that they render. In the past, health care professionals have traditionally been governed from within their professions. Decision making has become more complex as the rules and regulations require increasingly more external review, peer review, and involvement of other health team members, families, and clients in the health care decision-making arena. These are only a few examples of the real world of nursing practice; they are part of the nurse's everyday clinical decision making.

Since I became interested in bioethics in 1976, I have been immersed in the field. It has been a challenge to develop appropriate methods and strategies for teaching undergraduate and graduate students ethics in nursing and ethics in health care. At the University of South Florida College of Nursing, all undergraduate students are required to take a two-semester-hour course in Ethical-Legal Aspects in Nursing, and an Ethics in Health Care course is an elective offering for graduate students.

GUIDELINES FOR TEACHING ETHICS IN NURSING

This paper will present selected guidelines that were developed in the course of preparing *Teaching Ethics in Nursing* and *Case Studies for Students*.[1] These guidelines cover the following areas: (1) preparation of nursing faculty for teaching ethics, (2) student prerequisites for using the case study approach, (3) role and preparation of nurse ethicists in the health care setting, (4) development of a course outline, (5) techniques for implementing the case study approach, and (6) selected ethical issues in nursing.

Preparation of Nursing Faculty

The nurse educator's preparation for teaching ethics should include:

1. Basic knowledge of philosophical concepts, including moral philosophy, philosophical frameworks, philosophical principles and concepts, and ethical decision making.
2. Knowledge of contemporary ethical and legal issues affecting nurses as health care providers.
3. Knowledge of contemporary literature related to bioethics and issues in health care.
4. Identification of resource people within and outside of the educational setting.
5. Pursuit of educational activities, both formal and informal, such as seminars, workshops, discussion sessions, and fellowships related to ethics in health care.

---

[1] Minerva I. Applegate and Nina M. Entrekin, *Teaching Ethics in Nursing: A Handbook for Use of the Case-Study Approach* and *Case Studies for Students: A Companion to Teaching Ethics in Nursing* (New York: National League for Nursing, both 1984).

Student Prerequisites

Certain prerequisites must be considered before enrolling a student in a bioethics course. These are the following:

1. An introduction to terminology.
2. An introduction to philosophical frameworks.
3. A beginning knowledge of principles of ethical decision making.
4. An awareness of the literature sources.
5. An understanding of the roles of health team members.
6. A knowledge of communication systems within the health care system.
7. An understanding of hospital policies and procedures.
8. Comprehension of the relationship between legal and ethical considerations of nursing practice.
9. An understanding of the relationship between accountability and autonomy.

These prerequisites, as indicated, include substantive knowledge that students would generally not possess upon entering the undergraduate nursing program. At that point, students generally have a limited knowledge of systems, although they may be aware of legal and ethical principles that have been inculcated in them over their lifetime. At the present time, there appears to be little difference in the knowledge base of students at the undergraduate and graduate levels in nursing as related to bioethical theories, concepts, and principles. Graduate students ask the same type of questions as undergraduate students, and all the students seem to be searching for answers to difficult questions. One major difference is that the undergraduate students have limited experience in clinical practice. As soon as they enter the practice setting, however, they begin asking questions based on their observations and experiences, and many of these questions have ethical overtones. Students soon become familiar with a variety of ethical and legal concerns in nursing practice. Students need specific preparation prior to entering a course in bioethics if the experience is to be meaningful.

Role and Preparation of the Nurse Ethicist

The role of the nurse ethicist in health care is to:

1. Serve as a resource person in education, service, and research.
2. Disseminate information regarding ethical-legal issues and problems that nurses encounter in clinical practice through research and publications.

3. Organize ethics groups within education and practice settings.

4. Plan seminars and workshops to promote multidisciplinary awareness of ethical concerns in health care.

5. Promote the integration of bioethical principles and concepts as part of the preparation for professional nursing practice.

The nurse ethicist role requires the following preparation:

1. Undergraduate and graduate courses in philosophy of education, philosophy of science, bioethics, logic, social policy, legal aspects of health care, moral philosophy, medical ethics, and nursing ethics.

2. Affiliation with nursing colleagues who are aware of contemporary ethical and legal issues affecting nursing practice.

3. Affiliation with ethicists for exploration and didactic discussion of ethical issues and problems in health care from a multidisciplinary perspective.

4. Acquisition of a beginning personal library of literature resources such as classic philosophy books, bioethics books, encyclopedias, bibliographies, and journal subscriptions to selected bioethics publications.

5. Familiarity with contemporary legal and ethical issues affecting health care delivery; knowledge of pro and con arguments presented in the literature on each issue. The positions of major bioethicists on these issues should be identified and readily available to the nurse ethicist.

6. Clear identification of the nurse ethicist's philosophical position on contemporary ethical and legal issues.

Course Outline

Based on past experience, I would recommend the following as a basic outline for course content when teaching ethics in nursing:

1. Ethical theories, concepts, and principles.

2. Moral reasoning and values clarification.

3. Contemporary ethical issues.

4. Standards that guide nursing practice, including the Code for Nurses, Standards of Nursing Practice, Patients' Bill of Rights, and nurse practice acts.

5. Group presentations and discussions.

6. Case study presentations and discussions.

7. Panel discussions.

8. Review of course objectives and content.

9. (For courses on the master's level) Session on teaching ethics in nursing—the affective domain.

Assuming that a course in ethics in nursing would be taught over 15 sessions, one probably should plan to spend at least 3 sessions on theory. For undergraduate students, one could combine the legal and ethical aspects within the theory presentations. Graduate students should enter the program possessing knowledge of the basic legal principles and concepts that underlie professional nursing practice. Therefore, the primary focus in teaching ethics to graduate students should be on the development of substantive knowledge related to ethics in health care. Ethical theories, concepts, and principles should be introduced early on so that students can use this knowledge throughout the course. Values clarification and moral reasoning are two other content areas that should be introduced early in the course. Students should be introduced to contemporary ethical and legal issues in nursing practice and health care.[2]

The standards that guide nursing practice should be reviewed, including the American Nurses' Association's Code for Nurses (1976) and Standards for Nursing Practice (1973). The American Hospital Association's Patient's Bill of Rights (1972) and the state's nurse practice act should also be covered. All these documents serve to establish the ethical and legal parameters for professional nursing practice. Surprisingly, even graduate students are not familiar with the nurse practice acts that govern their nursing practice. Very few nurses are able to identify all the components of the documents that guide the ethical and legal parameters of nursing practice.

Case Study Approach

One effective method of teaching ethics in nursing is the use of case studies. This method is effective for both undergraduate and graduate nursing students. The following techniques are successful when used in conjunction with the case study approach:

1. Small-group discussion
2. Role playing
3. Use of audiovisuals
4. Debate
5. Panels of experts
6. Study questions

---

[2] Terry Pence, *Ethics in Nursing: An Annotated Bibliography* (New York: National League for Nursing 1983; 2nd. ed. in press).

7. Field experiences

8. Student presentations[3]

An effective way to demonstrate the process of multidisciplinary philosophical discourse at the end of the course is to arrange a panel discussion with a group of experts in bioethics. An appropriate topic is chosen for discussion, and the course instructor sends advance materials to each panel member. The instructor serves as a moderator, facilitator, and participant. Following the panel discussion, students may ask questions of the presenters, or they may engage in a discussion related to the topic. This type of presentation lends itself to videotaping, and the outcome may be that of an excellent teaching resource for future classes.

All students participate in group presentations related to a topic of their interest. In addition, students are required to write a scholarly paper in an area of interest, and an annotated bibliography is submitted with this paper.

Selected Ethical Issues

The basic ethical issues to be presented in an ethics in nursing or health care course are clearly identified in Pence's annotated bibliography, *Ethics in Nursing*.[4] This volume, which is a recommended textbook for all students in our ethics in nursing course, surveys 75 years of nursing literature in regard to ethical issues. We use a case study approach to teach ethics in nursing at the undergraduate level and recommend as a handbook for students *Case Studies for Students*.[5] Any of several nursing ethics books that have recently been published could be used as a required or supplementary textbook.[6] Reich's *Encyclopedia of Bioethics* and Walters' *Bibliography of Bioethics* make excellent reference sources.[7]

THE EVOLVING ETHICS COURSE

Over the past nine years, I have taught ethics in nursing to a variety of students. Every course seems to evolve in a different way, according to "where the students are at." In some of the courses, students tend to focus on easily identified issues such as abortion, euthanasia, and suicide. At other times, the focus has been more complex and global, fo-

---

[3] Applegate and Entrekin, *Case Studies for Students*.

[4] Pence, *Ethics in Nursing*.

[5] Applegate and Entrekin, *Case Studies for Students*.

[6] *See*, for example, J. E. Thompson and H. O. Thompson, *Bioethical Decision Making for Nurses* (Norwalk, Conn.: Appleton-Century-Crofts, 1985); K. M. Fenner, *Ethics and Law in Nursing: Professional Perspectives* (New York: D. Van Nostrand Co., 1980); and M. Benjamin and J. Curtis, *Ethics in Nursing* (New York: Oxford University Press, 1981).

[7] Warren T. Reich, *Encyclopedia of Bioethics*, 4 vols. (New York: Macmillan Publishing Co., 1978); and Leroy Walters, ed., *Bibliography of Bioethics*, Vol. 10 (New York: Macmillan Publishing Co., 1984).

cusing on topics such as the health care provider's rights, patients' rights, truth, and human experimentation or on humanistic concerns, such as the role of hospice nurses in caring for the terminally ill or dying patient. Group sizes have ranged from 12 to 70 students. Guest speakers have been varied, from transplant coordinators to genetic counselors. One new objective recently added to the graduate course addressed the acquisition of skills for teaching ethics in nursing.

As the class size has grown, new strategies have been implemented. For example, one semester when the class had 70 undergraduate students, four nursing faculty with preparation in ethics served as facilitators for small-group discussions and case analyses following presentations and discussions with the larger group.

The suggested techniques for implementing the case study approach have been used successfully many times at the University of South Florida. Given the opportunity, students can be extremely creative. Small-group sessions afford opportunities for values clarification and in-depth exploration of issues. Role-playing is very effective, and it gives students an opportunity to practice new decision-making skills. Audiovisuals can also be effective, and this type of class lends itself to the development of audiovisual materials, particularly videotaping. Debates afford the students an opportunity to practice techniques of argumentation. Students are extremely adept at finding "experts" for class presentations or discussions. Field experiences lend a sense of reality to very critical issues, and these experiences can be shared. Student presentations are generally creative and thought provoking.

In summary, before undertaking the teaching of ethics in nursing, one has to give careful consideration to the prerequisite substantive knowledge for both faculty and students. A variety of instructional strategies may be used effectively to enhance students' abilities to think critically and to foster systematic ethical decision making. The faculty member needs to be aware of resources (literature, media, and individuals) prior to undertaking the teaching of ethics. An environment of acceptance and flexibility must be provided for the students. The outcomes of the teaching experience are positive, and these outcomes can be measured in the cognitive as well as the affective domain.

An example of a course outline for teaching ethics appears in Figure 1. Recognition is given to the need for diversity among course offerings according to needs and priorities. This outline is offered merely as a frame of reference in the curriculum development process. Courses may differ according to levels and time frames. The outcomes, however, will probably be the same: nurses who are more humanistic and better prepared to engage in ethical decision making within the context of nursing and health care. The ultimate outcome may be improved patient care.

Figure 1. Proposed Course Syllabus for Ethical-Legal Aspects in Nursing and Health Care

Credits: Two (2) semester hours

Purpose: To introduce the student to contemporary bioethical and legal issues confronting health care providers in a variety of settings. The major focus of the course will be on ethical decision making and the identification of the legal and ethical parameters associated with contemporary nursing practice.

Objectives: The learner will:
1. Demonstrate comprehension of the major ethical theories influencing ethical decision making.
2. Identify the steps of a selected ethical decision-making model.
3. Identify ethical principles that enter into the ethical decision-making process.
4. Identify legal principles that must be considered when making decisions in health care.
5. Identify contemporary legal and ethical issues that are confronting health care providers.
6. Apply legal-ethical principles in hypothetical situations confronting health care providers.
7. Analyze hypothetical situations in health care that have ethical and legal implications for nurses as health care providers.
8. Actively participate in class discussions and presentations related to ethical and legal decisions in health care.
9. Demonstrate synthesis of knowledge through submission of a scholarly paper that focuses on a contemporary legal-ethical issue in health care.

Evaluation:
1. Group presentation—25%
2. Written issues paper—50%
3. Annotated bibliography—25%

Guidelines for Written Analysis:
1. Select an ethical issue and identify the issue within the framework of contemporary health care.
2. State your position as related to the ethical issue.
3. Review the literature as it relates to the selected issue. Present more than one viewpoint on the issue.
4. Identify the implications of the issue for health care providers.
5. State your conclusions and recommendations.
6. Adhere to scholarly principles.

Guidelines for Seminar Discussion:
1. Submit analysis of issue at least two weeks prior to discussion session.
2. Demonstrate adequate preparation for discussion of selected issue, including:
   A. Knowledge of basic theoretical framework from which issue may be viewed.
   B. Knowledge of various positions taken by authors in the literature.
   C. Consideration of the implications for health care providers.
   D. Logical and orderly presentation of the issue.
3. Facilitate learning through the appropriate utilization of principles of group process, including clarification, feedback, validation, and summarization.
4. Consider time limits and allow time to summarize discussion and achieve closure.

Guidelines for Annotated Bibliography: Entries are to include:
1. Identification of reading with appropriate citation.
2. Identification of purpose/objectives of author.
3. Identification of theoretical framework/major focus of reading.
4. Identification of methodology, sample, instrument, data collection, and data analysis, if appropriate.
5. Conclusions, recommendations, and implications for health care providers.

CHANGE, CHALLENGES, AND COALITIONS: KALEIDOSCOPE OF NURSING AND VOCATIONAL EDUCATION

DORA B. JOHNSON, EdD, RN
President, The Baldwin Center
Greeley, Colorado

Nursing and vocational education are a historical team. Practical nursing programs have received vocational education funds since the Smith-Hughes Act in 1917. Then, in 1956, Title III of the George Barden Act specifically authorized expenditure of funds for practical nursing education. In the Vocational Educational Act of 1964, eligibility was expanded to any program providing education below the level of the baccalaureate degree; this is where associate degree nursing programs first received their vocational education funds. The *Fact Sheet* on health occupations education (HOE) in area-vocational schools reports that "the most frequently reported HOE program in area-vocational schools is Practical Nursing with 10 states reporting secondary programs and 20 states reporting postsecondary programs."[1] Vocational education represents the single largest funding source for nursing programs in the United States. We must continue to develop the team of nursing and vocational education.

The state of nursing and vocational education resembles a kaleidoscope. The bits of colored glass make geometric designs, but the minute

---

[1] Lauretta Cole, ed., *American Vocational Association Fact Sheet—Health Occupations Education in United States Area-Vocational Schools* (Arlington, Va.: American Vocational Association, 1985).

the tube is jiggled or turned, the picture changes. We are looking through a giant kaleidoscope right now in nursing and vocational education, but we must do more than just look. Changes, challenges, and coalitions require us to act.

CHANGES

A list of the changes in nursing that have occurred in the past 5, 10, or 20 years would be exceptionally long. Let me review a few and add some that may not have been considered.

Until a few years ago, the wisdom was that "a nurse can always get a job." Therefore, we could leave work and take time to raise children. We would need refresher courses but could always get back into the nursing work force. This is no longer so.

Until a few years ago, all nursing programs were overenrolled. There were waiting lists. We could screen out candidates, hold lotteries for the slots, prescribe numerous entrance requirements, and admit extra students to allow for attrition. This is no longer so.

Until a few years ago, nurses in hospitals and nursing homes could provide nursing care to each patient without being overly concerned about the overall operation of the facility. Only when a nurse moved into management did budget and cost containment become a daily concern. This is no longer so.

Until a few years ago, vocational education also had many students, so we did not have to worry about jobs. We also had waiting lists and did not need to be overly concerned with costs. In addition to changes in these areas, there has been the shift in educational emphasis. However, all the documents about quality in education barely mention vocational education and then only in a limited or negative fashion. In the public concern for education, vocational education does not receive a high priority for school district funds. The atmosphere in which vocational education prospered also no longer exists.

In the health care field there have been radical changes. As Brown notes, in the 1940s and 1950s there was subsidization; in the 1960s and 1970s regulation; and now, in the 1980s, there is competition.[2] She goes on to identify changes in acute care, including:

- Shift to outpatient services
- Increase in write-offs
- Efforts to decrease overhead
- Continued decrease in length of stay

---

[2] Lynn Brown, "Trends in Health Care" (Greeley: North Colorado Medical Center, 1985).

- Continued increase in high technology
- Continued decrease in admissions
- Increased acuity of patients
- Emphasis on increased productivity
- Greater difficulty in obtaining capital dollars
- Shift from revenue control approach
- Cost-accounting measures
- Reimbursement changes
- Diversification
- Integration of related services
- Expanded service areas

Until a few years ago, every town had its hospital, even if it had only five acute-care beds and the remaining were for long-term care. This is no longer so. In fact, Ellwood, a health policy researcher and president of InterStudy, predicts that in 10 years there will be only 20 companies providing health care services in the United States.[3] He contends that the 300,000 hospitals, insurance plans, prepaid practices, and medical groups in existence today will be operated by these 20 national firms by 1995. These firms will include three insurers, two Blue Cross or Blue Shield plans, two proprietary hospital chains, two nonprofit hospital groups, one Kaiser plan, two health maintenance organizations, two academic medical centers, two multispeciality groups, and three others—"maybe a Sears Roebuck or something along that line."

In an earlier period of history, our society moved from a farming to an industrial society. That society no longer exists as we move into the information society described in *Megatrends*.[4] Many other shifts follow as part of that information society: from forced technology to "high technology/high touch," from nation to world, from short term to long term, from institution to self, from hierarchies to networks, and from either-or to multiple options.

Change is all around nursing and vocational education—not only within the organizations where we work, but throughout the entire world. This phenomenon of constant change is like a paint pot—the colorful, mudlike hot springs in Yellowstone National Park. The pot is constantly moving, with bubbles coming to the surface periodically and bursting. When each bubble breaks, it adds a color, which is swirled by the movement into the rest of the pot. This new color gradually fades until it becomes indis-

---

[3] Paul Ellwood, Jr., "Big Firms to Dominate Health Care," *Allied Health Education Newsletter* (1985).

[4] John Naisbitt, *Megatrends: Ten New Directions Transforming Our Lives* (New York: Warner Books, 1982).

tinguishable from all the other colors, yet the pot is now somewhat different.

Nursing and vocational education are in the middle of change. We can continue to look through the kaleidoscope, admiring the changing colors, patterns, and highlights. Or we can take the risk and become involved in that paint pot with its constantly changing colors, motion, and outcomes. Nursing leaders can make practical and associate degree nursing a vital part of all these changes; however, with leadership come challenges.

CHALLENGES

It has been said that people do not have problems—rather, we encounter challenges. Thus, the changes just outlined can be viewed in terms of challenges that we can put to use in nursing and vocational education.

Accepting Change

I challenge nursing to truly accept that health care is and will be different from what it was in the past. Growth involves trade-offs. Adding a service will mean dropping something else or lowering the price so that both are affordable. Health services will be in competition with all budget items, so that consumers will shop competitively for health care just as they now do for clothing or food. The future of health care is uncertain at best. Therefore, past trends are irrelevant and new trends are unknown or changing. Just when a new trend is in focus it will move. Bauer, a health economist, outlines some of the factors that will affect the future of health care and forecasts their effects, among them, the following:

- Deinstitutionalization will produce rapid movement away from hospital-centered health care systems.
- The change from one level of quality to differing levels of quality in care will result in a variety of types of services.
- The increasing imperative for efficiency will result in least-cost production.
- A prolonged period in which there is a surplus of physicians will make interprofessional division more bitter.
- Attention to effectiveness will lead to the rejection of unproductive programs.
- Healthier people will mean a decline in the incidence of preventable conditions.[5]

---

[5] Jeffry C. Bauer, "Strategic Planning Today for Health Care Programs Tomorrow," paper presented at a meeting of Long's Peak Association of Occupational Health Nurses, Longmont, Colorado, March 1984.

We cannot continue to wait for the "good old days" to return—they will not. The challenge is to accept that health care has changed and will continue to change. What can we do? Let me propose a few suggestions.

I challenge nursing education to change its curriculum. Include job opportunities for entrepreneurs, not just employment in hospitals or nursing homes; provide clinical experience in walk-in clinics, home care, and private industry; concentrate on concepts, generalizations, and principles for easier transfer to new situations.

Becoming Involved

I challenge nurse educators to become involved in the vocational education system and professional association in their state. Vocational education has new federal legislation, the Carl D. Perkins Vocational Education Act of 1984.[6] There are some critical changes in purposes of this legislation that affect nursing programs. The following are some examples:

> Purpose A. Assist the States to expand, improve, modernize and develop quality vocational education programs to meet needs of existing and future work force. . . .

No longer can federal funds be used to fund ongoing, unchanging programs. Funds can be allocated, however, to *expand*, *improve*, and *modernize*, and I am sure that all programs have areas that can be expanded, improved, or modernized. Those who are aware of this legislation can contact their state vocational agency to order the proposal guidelines or find out the procedure to tap into those funds for their program.

> Purpose D. Improve academic foundations and to aid in application of newer technologies (including computers). . . .

Nursing certainly has a science base that has not been readily identified by others. What better way to demonstrate the academic foundations than to outline the science competencies found in nursing programs or to propose computer applications in health care that would also provide in-school computer experience for students?

> Purpose E. Provide services to train, retrain, and upgrade . . . in new skills. . . .

---

[6] P. L. 98-524, *Carl D. Perkins Vocational Education Act* (Washington, D.C.: U.S. Government Printing Office, 1984).

This item is a clear signal for the provision of adult and continuing education in the health care field. Every school should be able to offer several short-term classes to provide retraining or upgrading.

There are nine purposes in the new act. Each one has an impact on nursing programs and provides possibilities for them. Nurse educators must be in contact with other vocational educators so that they can be informed when such changes come about.

Nursing Education as a Business

I challenge nurse educators to consider their programs as a business. According to the Small Business Administration, if you agree with eight or more of the following statements, "you probably have what it takes to run a business."

- I do things on my own. Nobody has to tell me to get going.
- I like people. I can get along with just about anybody.
- I can get most people to go along when I start something.
- I like to take charge of things and see them through.
- I like to have a plan before I start. I'm usually the one to get things lined up when the group wants to do something.
- I can keep going as long as I need to. I don't mind working hard for something I want.
- I can make up my mind in a hurry if I have to. It usually turns out OK, too.
- People can trust me. I don't say things I don't mean.
- If I make up my mind to do something. I don't let anything stop me.
- I never run down.[7]

The literature suggests that in the future small business will grow most rapidly, while the large corporations will not do as well.

Among the characteristics of excellent businesses identified by Peters and Waterman is a bias for action.[8] The people running these businesses don't talk about doing something, they do it. How many times have we in nursing talked about an issue—and talked and talked? I challenge nurse educators to act. You can't plow a field by turning it over in your mind. You won't always be right, but as John Henry Newman said, "Noth-

---

[7] *Checklist for Going into Business* (Forth Worth, Tex.: Small Business Administration, n.d.).

[8] Thomas J. Peters and Robert H. Waterman, Jr., *In Search of Excellence—Lessons from America's Best-Run Companies* (New York: Harper & Row, 1982).

ing would be done if a man waited until he could do it so well that no one could find fault with it."

According to Peters and Waterman, excellent companies also keep close to the customer. Nursing education's customers are students and the employers who hire its graduates. The advisory committee that represents all facets of a program and its customers has been one of vocational education's strengths. I challenge programs that do not have such a group to develop one.

Staying Aware

I challenge nurse educators to pay attention to all segments of the communities in which they live and work. The current atmosphere has been described as multidimensional—one in which vertical systems or single-dimensional plans will not work. The society within which we, our programs, vocational education, and health care operate is constantly changing. To keep current, we must be aware of any slight changes. We must also be sensitive if we expect to have an impact on that society. We must be aware of the unique characteristics of the communities in which our programs are located and where our students are hired.

Each piece of information is critical. For example, a consulting group was trying to overcome community resistance to a large recreational area being located next to their town. They considered the patterns of the town and discovered that in one community there was a post office that refused to deliver. Therefore, everyone in that community had to come in contact with the postmaster everyday. The group made sure that the postmaster was fully informed about their project and that written information was readily available in the post office. In the other community, they discovered that the town butcher was outstanding, so everyone bought their meat from him. Again, they made sure that the butcher was informed. These activities were in addition to numerous other developmental activities, but it was this multidimensional approach that made the difference. Just going through the town council would not have worked.

Thus, nurse educators must consider what patterns they must be aware of within the clinical agencies they use. When you want to develop change in one student, which one of the other students might be influential? In your school, whom must you alert about your plans? Many times the answers to these questions do not fall within the formal system structure of the organization you are attempting to influence.

Now, how can we possibly identify and keep track of all this information? The answer is that we do not have to be personally aware of all the patterns—we can involve others. Through networks and coalitions we exponentially increase our ability to gather information or influence decisions.

COALITIONS

Because of the information overload, it is not possible for a single person to have all the information on a particular subject. In addition, it is not possible to contact all parties who would be interested in a particular topic. This is where networks and coalitions come into play and become a critical part of the kaleidoscope.

We are not only changing from an industrial to an informational society, but we are also changing from hierarchies to networks in order to achieve outcomes.[9] We are beginning to recognize that pyramids within organizations and management will not solve problems. The speed of the telephone, airplane, and computer requires that we respond rapidly. Information is a great equalizer; and the network, which is informal and equal, where communication is both lateral and diagonal, is becoming the method by which information is gathered so that decisions can be made.

A picture of a network would look like a spiderweb. It starts at the center and goes in all directions. Some strands are long and some short, some thick and some thin. All parts are connected, however, and any part of the web can be reached from any other part. Networks are people webs. People are at the center, joined by local, state, national, and international connections made through business, family, friends, business friends, and a myriad of other associations. All parts are connected, and it is possible to contact anyone by using the web of people in the network.

Each person's contacts are different and spin in different directions. A coalition is simply a temporary alliance between people, factions, or organizations. The coalition is generated because of networking, and once the task for the coalition is complete, the people involved once again become simply a part of the network.

Nursing education has not developed adequate networks and coalitions to assist in what it wishes to do. Nurse educators have been talking among themselves too much, instead of talking with other groups and thereby expanding their networks and scope of possible impact. There are two ways to approach building a network. We can identify something we want, such as travel money for students to attend a state or national organization, scholarships, or a donation of equipment. But frequently we eliminate possible connections because we are not able to visualize their potential. The second approach is to contact organizations before a need arises to explore possibilities that could mean many more opportunities than we might have identified initially. If you go to an organization with only one idea, that is probably all you will come away with.

Why not decide to contact one organization per month. Meet with some-

---

[9] Naisbitt, *Megatrends.*

169

one from the organization to explore possibilities of working together. Be sure to go into that meeting with an open mind and listen to what the other person is saying about that organization's health care needs. Don't leave the meeting, however, until there is some action you and the other organization are willing to take—even if it is only to meet again in three months to consider other possibilities. Identify other organizations to contact so that your coalition continues to increase in its number and scope. No other field besides health affects every person; therefore a connection can be established with every organization. Some examples for coalitions might include working with the following groups:

- The local chamber of commerce to set up CPR training for businesses. Your school of nursing might help as a way to let students teach and practice their skills. The chamber of commerce could agree to have each business survey their employees to determine personal or family interest in nursing programs—a source of possible recruits.

- Unions to initiate a stress assessment and prevention program or breast or prostate self-examination, which students could use as patient education projects. The union could in turn agree to sponsor one of the students to attend a meeting of the state or national Health Occupations Students of America.

- The local dental society to arrange a presentation at one of their meetings on how consumer health is affecting nursing care. The society could agree to assist in working for legislation relating to the state nursing practice act.

- The county agriculture agent to work with local farmers on farm first aid as a community project for the student organization. In return, the agent could include in his or her next newsletter information about a local issue of vital interest, such as a request for an increased budget.

The major reason that people do not join professional associations is that no one ever asks them. Many groups, organizations, agencies, and departments would work with nursing programs in some capacity if we just asked them.

I know that nursing educators have limited time to make such contacts because they are very much involved in teaching, administering, supervising, and evaluating. But we must use our network. Just think how much could be accomplished if everyone on the nursing program staff agreed to use his or her network and develop one organizational contact in a year. Don't play the superperson and believe that you have to do all of it yourself—that's not how networks and coalitions work most effectively. When everyone is involved, when everyone has responsibility, when everyone has equal risk in creating something new and exciting, that is when the network and coalition are most effective.

There is already a coalition between nursing and vocational education. The Health Occupations Division of the American Vocational Association and the Association itself have repeatedly supported practical and associate degree nursing. The National Advisory Council on Vocational Education supports levels of nursing.[10] Vocational education organizations and agencies within each state also offer support. The connection between us is already there. What must be done now is to increase the numbers of organizations involved.

CONCLUSION

There have been many changes in nursing but with changes have come new possibilities we would not have considered a few years ago. There are challenges, because with change there are new ways of working together with which we are not familiar. We are therefore afraid of failure. But to assist with both, there are networks and coalitions—there are people. We are in the middle of the paint pot and it is bubbling.

Dr. Johnson may be contacted at The Baldwin Center, 1623 14th Ave., Greeley, Co. 80631, (303) 356-0065.

---

[10] *The Education of Nurses—A Rising National Concern*, Issue Paper No. 2 (Washington, D.C.: National Advisory Council on Vocational Education, 1980).

political and economic aspects of nursing

ANALYZING THE EFFECTS OF PROSPECTIVE PAYMENT: QUESTIONS FOR NURSING

MARY KAYE WILLIAN, DrPH, RN
Health Policy Analyst
Prospective Payment Assessment Commission
Washington, D.C.

In writing the original 1983 prospective payment legislation, Congress, in all its wisdom, recognized the important role that nursing plays in the delivery of care. This recognition was again apparent in a recently introduced bill to expand the membership of the Prospective Payment Assessment Commission (ProPAC), which stated that, with respect to nursing services:

> It goes without saying that the input of nursing will be essential in any attempt to make the payment system relevant to the care being provided in hospitals. Nurses remain a primary source of direct patient care in hospitals and, on average, spend more time than any other group with hospital inpatients.[1]

This recognition speaks to the concern of Congress that the prospective payment system may adversely affect quality of services and access to care for Medicare beneficiaries. This concern was, in part, the reason for the establishment of ProPAC. At the beginning of 1984, there were alarming predictions that hospital work forces would be reduced, nurses would

---

[1] Senate Bill 984, *Congressional Record*, April 24, 1985, S4687.

be fired, Medicare beneficiaries would be thrown out of hospitals, and those patients remaining in the hospital would receive less than adequate care.

WHAT IS HAPPENING TO HEALTH CARE?

A recent article in the *Wall Street Journal* addressed the issue of the effects of prospective payment on quality of care.[2] The article commented on a letter that was printed in Ann Landers' column from a medical student complaining about nurses' attitudes. Nursing's response to this letter was, according to Ann Landers, "staggering." She received 7,000 letters outlining the mounting difficulties for a profession already known for long hours and low pay. Nurses cited instances of exhaustion and stress so severe that patients' lives were endangered. Ann Landers is quoted as saying that it is the most depressing mail she has read in years.

The *Wall Street Journal* cited Medicare's new payment system as one of the major causes of hospitals' move to reduce nursing and support staffs. A health care analyst at Ernst and Whinney was quoted as saying that "the nurse is where the buck can't be passed any more. They [nurses] are the biggest victims of cost-cutting because they can't hide from the patient."

The article cited examples of deteriorations in quality of nursing services such as inappropriate reductions in frequency of suctioning patients; orders for medications, procedures, and dressing changes left for the next shift; and failure to walk a patient who needs to be walked several times a day. Some of the situations cited were life-threatening; others prolonged length of hospital stay or decreased the likelihood that individuals would return to their optimal states of functioning.

It is easy to become incensed reading such articles. What is happening to one of the best, if not the best, health care system in the world? Have we taken our cost-containment activities too far?

The honest response to this question is that we just do not know. I recently heard a nurse tell an audience that the initials *D-R-G* stand not for "diagnosis related groups" but rather for "dead, recovered, or gone." I hope that we can be more optimistic about the new payment system. We know it has flaws. The health care system is in a state of tremendous transition. Prospective payment is new, and we need some time to see how it will work out.

No one would deny that cost-based reimbursement was a fairly fat system, and nurses were part of that fat. In many places, the health care

---

[2] "Hospital Nightmare: Cuts in Staff Demoralize Nurses as Care Suffers," *Wall Street Journal*, March 27, 1985.

system was like Topsy—it just grew. There was not really a planned strategy. We reacted to the need for care—perceived or real—it is hard to know which. But those days are over now. We have stopped being reactors and have become thinkers and planners. We are now striving for a leaner system, the challenge being to determine just how lean we can become without damaging the components of care treasured so highly in this country—those of quality and access.

Nurses are in key positions to guide the health care system into the future, and educators and academicians can bridge the gap between academia and service by bringing anecdotal and clinical information to the realm of research analysis. This is what is needed to answer many of the policy-related questions that are being asked in Washington these days.

NURSING ISSUES AT PROPAC

By statute, ProPAC is required to look at the quality of health care provided in hospitals, including the quality and skill level of professional nursing required to maintain quality of care. This mandate could be interpreted in a variety of ways, and ProPAC has no magical formula for how to measure quality. We are struggling with this issue just like everyone else.

As a first attempt, ProPAC has chosen to review how Medicare pays for nursing services. The hypothesis is that unless hospitals are paid appropriately for care provided, services to Medicare beneficiaries may be reduced or denied. To summarize the issue briefly, Medicare's method of allocating nursing costs is on a per diem basis, which implicitly assumes that costs are approximately the same among DRGs and that they do not vary by patient diagnosis and need for care. Anyone who has worked in a clinical setting knows this just is not so.

Because of Medicare's method of accounting for nursing services, there may be significant inaccuracies in the DRG weights on which payments to hospitals are based. As a result, there may be overpayment for some diagnoses and underpayment for others. Depending on the types of patients the hospital serves, some institutions may suffer losses, while others will make undeserved profits. This is an important equity problem both for Medicare beneficiaries and hospitals serving them. Hospitals, facing distorted incentives, may respond by either limiting admissions of patients with more costly conditions or reducing services to these individuals.

ProPAC also suspects that if we adjust the DRG system for nursing use, it may reduce the need for further modifications to the system for severity of illness. The commission will be looking into this problem. We view it as a priority area and have asked Secretary of Health and Human Services Margaret Heckler to devote resources to this issue as well.

177

The following are some of the questions with which ProPAC is currently struggling in relation to this project:

- What should be the basis of measurement for nursing intensity—the ICD-9 (International Classification of Diseases, ninth revision) diagnosis level; the major diagnostic category levels (MDCs) of the DRG system; or the DRG level?

- What approaches are reasonable to consider for costing nursing services? Is the per diem method, on average, okay? The commission does not think so, but as scientists we must ask and examine further this question. Would some form of a cost-to-charge ratio work? Or, should the method be patient- or diagnosis-focused like the DRG system?

- How should an adjustment for nursing services be incorporated into the national payment rates? Should it be a one-time only adjustment, or should it be done periodically to update the system for changes in the pattern of practice? If it should be updated, how frequently?

- If nursing costs are unbundled from the per diem, how should the remaining components of the per diem be handled?

When the commission began looking into this topic and seeking out studies regarding assessment of nursing resource use, we found few in the literature. Those that are available are limited in either the number of hospitals or DRGs included in the sample. We have a lot of work to do, and we are beginning at square one. It is an exciting area with which to be involved, and one the commission has deemed to be of major importance.

The nursing issue alone raises numerous important research topics that have policy implications and are of major significance to the health care system. Those in nursing education can become involved in these and other issues either by researching these topics themselves or stimulating their students to investigate them. Nurses have the capability to become important players in policy-related and health services research.

COSTING OUT NURSING EDUCATION: DILEMMA FOR NURSING SCHOOLS AND NURSING SERVICES

COLLEEN CONWAY-WELCH, PhD, CNM, FAAN
Professor and Dean
School of Nursing
Vanderbilt University
Nashville, Tennessee

The dilemma of "costing out" and paying for nursing education is of rising concern to educators, students, and consumers. Medicine and nursing are grappling with the need to identify the specific costs of undergraduate nursing and basic medical education as well as the specific costs of graduate nursing and graduate medical education.

Since the emergence of private and public insurers as the predominant payers of health care, financial support for undergraduate and graduate medical education has been viewed partially as a community responsibility. This is not so in the case of undergraduate and graduate nursing education. Today's third-party payers are also questioning the traditional practice of cross-subsidizing services deemed worthy by the community but not explicitly financed by it, such as care for the poor, regional standby services, and the education of health care professionals.

A 1985 report to the Association of Academic Health Centers, entitled *Out of the Temple and into the Marketplace*, emphasizes the new role of marketing in the entire health care arena, and the fact that academic health centers that educate physicians and nurses have special costs and needs. It notes that "Academic health care centers seem paralyzed to make the changes needed to cope with their marketing requirements."[1] Nursing education also shows signs of paralysis in coping with our marketing requirements as we face declining student enrollment, competition from the variety of attractive career choices available to women, and the interest of the federal government in reducing subsidies to health care educational programs in general.

COSTS OF NURSING EDUCATION

Nursing education itself is out of the temple and into the marketplace. Because diploma nursing programs are directly affected, nursing needs to be aware of education cost proposals currently before Congress and how these proposals attempt to address the cutbacks in Medicare pass-through funds, which have directly subsidized graduate medical education and diploma nursing programs for years. Associate degree, baccalaureate degree, and graduate degree programs are also vulnerable, because agencies have a strong interest in separating out the heretofore "hidden" costs of "clinical laboratories" for these students and in finding new sources of revenue to meet these costs. An increasing number of agencies are considering charging a "user fee" to schools of nursing if the agency is used as a clinical laboratory.

Arthur Young and Company is performing a cost-function analysis of graduate medical education in 44 hospitals for the Department of Health and Human Services Assistant Secretary for Planning and Evaluation. The Commonwealth Fund is sponsoring a similar analysis by the Center for Hospital Finance and Management. These analyses will be completed shortly. These reports do not address costs imposed by nursing education; the National League for Nursing (NLN) and the American Association of Colleges of Nursing (AACN) are addressing this issue. However, progress is slow due to lack of data and inconsistency among data.

The new word in health care—*competition*—is being promoted based on the *price* of care. Consumers are not necessarily interested in eliminating private and public support of health care for the poor and indigent and for expenses incurred by agencies as a result of teaching nursing and medical students. However, they want explicit government policies to finance these costs and therefore take them out of the patient care revenue stream that flows from patients' pockets and their insurance premiums.

Nurse educators must become active; we must work with federal and state agencies, legislators, and private agencies to explicitly identify the

---

[1] Barton-Gillet Co., *Out of the Temple and into the Marketplace* (Washington, D.C.: Association of Academic Health Centers, January 1985).

180

cost of the didactic and clinical components of nursing education and to develop new methods of paying for it. The results of the NLN and AACN studies will, we hope, provide guidelines for all of us to identify the costs of these components. For informed public policy about support for education for health care professionals, we need to know what the costs are and why they occur, and then assess the pros and cons of various funding mechanisms. As educators, we need to be active, not reactive. We must recognize the handwriting on the wall. We also need to track carefully what medicine is doing about this dilemma, because we are silent (or not-so-silent) partners with them in the solutions being considered and studied!

Before nurse educators can address the realistic concerns of nursing service and hospital administration over the nursing student portion of the costs of clinical education, we need to determine whether having nursing students in the clinical units is a net cost or a net benefit to an institution.

In addition, we frequently lack clarity about the actual costs of the didactic components of our education programs. Traditionally, didactic and clinical education in nursing has been financed by a mix of tuition and fees, federal and state grants and subsidies, private foundation money, and patient care revenues. In the past, schools used various settings for the clinical component, and financial arrangements were never mentioned because students were taught and supervised by nursing faculty. But today, hospitals are questioning the equity of this arrangement.

Frequently, the direct and indirect costs to a hospital or agency—and even to a school budget itself—have been vague and arguable. Determining the total costs of programs can be difficult. A school of nursing's accounting system may not have been established with this precise purpose in mind. The level of detail and number of cost centers in a school's budget have a significant impact on the ability to determine actual revenue and expenses associated with a specific academic unit, such as a department or a center for nursing research.

In his monograph, *Financial Analysis for Academic Units*, Walters makes the following points about determining these costs:

- Indirect as well as direct costs need to be measured.
- Cost has both fixed and variable elements in relation to the number of students or faculty in an academic unit.
- Revenue attributable to an academic unit needs to be measured.
- Costs per student full-time equivalent, per full-time equivalent faculty, and per class are all measures of a unit's cost.
- Weighted data is needed about the cost per student by level of study and method and setting of instruction.

- The expected cost of an academic unit can be determined by its level of average faculty and their workload. (However, given the manner in which most schools currently teach the clinical component, with wide variations in faculty time even in the same school, this can be very difficult.)
- Expenditure accounts listed in a unit's budget constitute the basis for determining only the unit's direct cost.[2]

Direct costs include salaries and benefits, consultants' fees, supplies and equipment, service contracts, telephone, postage, travel, duplicating and printing, and special "jobs" done for one unit by another unit. Indirect costs include salaries and benefits for people who provide services but are not assigned to the unit, utilities, and other expenses that supply support services. These can then be analyzed in terms of their variability (that is, the extent to which an increase or decrease in activity affects the costs, since "fixed" costs are insensitive to fluctuation).

A school can easily identify the salary costs of "regular" faculty. Estimating the indirect costs that students may impose on a hospital or agency budget because of staff nurse time spent with them is much more difficult to determine; these costs fall into the "variable" category.

ENROLLMENT AND TUITION

A major portion of many school's revenue projections depends on enrollment and tuition projections. In the past, with climbing or stable enrollments, the emphasis has been on how to project and meet these variable costs. With many schools facing decreasing enrollment, first variable costs and then fixed costs decrease, leading to sometimes painful decisions regarding faculty, staff, and space.

Trend-line analysis and financial modeling can be done once projections of enrollment, expenditures (direct and indirect costs), and revenue are in hand. We can then examine:

- The number and type of students needed for a sound fiscal plan.
- The number and type of faculty needed.
- The revenue and expenditures that vary according to enrollments.
- The need for increasing, decreasing, or retraining personnel.
- The kinds of plant facilities needed.
- The quantity and type of support services.

[2] D. L. Walters, *Financial Analysis for Academic Units*, Research Report No. 7 (Washington, D.C.: American Association for Higher Education, ERIC Clearinghouse on Higher Education, 1981).

- The strategies for winning *support* for changes in operations and programs resulting from changes in enrollment.

However, Walters cautions that equating cost alone to quality or fiscal efficiency to program effectiveness may result in disaster, since qualitative decisions must also be made.[3] A five-year revenue plan with a time line based on the cost-center concept, assigning revenue as well as cost to specific cost-centers, can help the nurse administrator to make some of these qualitative decisions.

The cost of tuition increases on a regular basis at a rate comparable with inflation. A major portion of most schools' revenue projections depends on enrollment and subsequent tuition projections. When faced with declining enrollment in the past, schools have chosen one of three courses of action—they either increased tuition, increased enrollment, or closed the program and reopened with a different mission and a new and reduced number of faculty and students.

With an increase in tuition, the school *must* increase available financial aid. At least 10 to 15 percent of tuition must be returned directly to students in a financial aid package; some schools return as much as 25 percent. This, of course, offsets the benefits to be gained by raising tuition. However, it is a marketing principle that a school should not be the cheapest in its category—students may then elect to go to a school that charges more because it "must be better"! With a successful increase in tuition, schools can initiate program changes that cut enrollment. The number of faculty can then be reduced by decreasing the number of regular faculty and by implementing dual appointments with service agencies and joint appointments with other schools on campus. In the latter instances, the agency or other school pays an agreed-on portion of the salary, encouraging faculty to engage in faculty practice activities. Achieving a successful increase in enrollment while holding tuition steady is more difficult. A school can increase its recruitment budget, but other schools will also be doing this.

The schools that will survive these troubled times are those in which the administrator of the nursing education unit controls her or his own budget. Only then can the school respond with needed changes and plans, and only then can the financial impact of these plans be modeled and implemented in a timely fashion.

Our ability to disregard the machinations of federal funding must also be increased. Historically, if federal money was available for something, we did it. Many schools used "soft" federal money for programs integral to the structure of the school, and many also started new programs with federal money and minimal curriculum and financial planning.

---

[3] *Ibid.*

183

THE CLINICAL COMPONENT

As schools and clinical agencies struggle with the issue of who pays for the clinical component of nursing education, the following areas must be considered:

- The nature of the clinical education (length and shift, intensity, and location).
- Current and possible organizational or contractual arrangements between programs and the institution.
- Services provided by the staff to the students.
- Services provided by the students to the staff and patients.
- Level of student.
- Physical availability of the faculty member to the student and the staff.
- The type and location of clinical settings used.

Historically, most health education was an apprenticeship in the agency; today it is primarily didactic, with the agency used as a "clinical laboratory." Hospitals started programs to provide a continuous core of personnel for their own institution, and they provided supervision and facilities to the students to achieve this goal. The "burying" of direct and indirect costs to the agency for the education of nursing and medical students has a long history. The shift from that of "sponsor" to that of "affiliate" is a recent one, as universities and two-year colleges started their own nursing education programs, and the didactic portion of the educational process became more distinct from the clinical portion.

As schools attempt to establish the cost for clinical education, both in and out of the hospital, the following statements should be recognized as "givens":

- The nature and level of teaching activity varies both among and within hospitals.
- Measures of teaching, faculty workloads, and staff workloads should reflect varying degrees of involvement in teaching.
- Differences in patient case mix need to be considered.

The degree to which nursing students can serve as substitutes or adjuncts for nursing staff is largely dependent on the content of the teaching program. It is thought that a major factor contributing to indirect cost of nursing education is the change in productivity levels of the staff. Studies have shown mixed results: students consume time but provide services; substitution of students for more expensive fully trained personnel may partially balance the loss in productivity resulting from their presence.

Today, there is no consensus on the overall cost of losses in productivity or the degree to which these losses are diluted by substitution effects. The old idea was to send in faculty so students would not affect staff. However, nurse educators know that this is a dead model—it is too expensive to send a large number of faculty into the "clinical laboratory." It is interesting to note that (1) the model of other sciences is that laboratory supervision is generally provided by teaching assistants who are usually graduate students; and (2) even in medicine, residents (graduate students) carry the major load of clinical teaching of medical students. Nursing, unlike medicine, social work, and psychology, for example, is the only profession that attempts to send our regular faculty into our institutions.

What is being proposed may be considered heresy, but a major change is needed. We must move away from the idea that the hospital (or other setting) is a "clinical laboratory." Schools of nursing can no longer afford to send in, on a full-time basis, "lab instructors" (faculty) who are not carrying their own patient or research loads and who are not generating a portion of their salaries.

Students are complaining. There is distrust between faculty and staff nurses. Why not send our students to clerkships and preceptorships where they would be paired with staff nurses in a variety of settings and use faculty in creative ways to validate the learning that is occurring, both on the part of the staff nurses and the student? These staff nurses are the graduate students and faculty of tomorrow—why not awaken them to the challenges and rewards of teaching? Why not use computer simulations for a larger portion of the learning process and use faculty to evaluate the student demonstrations that learning has occurred?

STRATEGIES FOR CHANGE

As we take a hard look at the cost of clinical education, strategies for change must be based on the facts that (1) we are currently facing a 25 percent reduction in size of traditional college-going population; and (2) the federal government will continue to be involved in nursing education (albeit on a much lower level) because educational programs do increase quality of health care; as a purchaser of health care, the federal government has some responsibility to share the cost; and special national needs will continue to exist.

In the next few years, it is likely that both private and public schools of nursing will seek state funds even more than federal funds for student aid and start-up funds for programs that address specific local needs. There are other things that schools can do.

If schools rely heavily on tuition, they must make program decisions that will either raise tuition and decrease expenses, or increase enrollment in specific programs. As numbers of students shrink, fresh viewpoints and more flexibility in nursing education programs will be necessary.

Schools need to move faster. There must be changes in programs and in delivery. In this electronic age, we have to recognize that decisive action must be taken—we cannot continue endlessly to meet and discuss, discuss and meet. Faculty committees need to be empowered to move—and one of the roles of successful deans will be that of empowering faculty. Financial modeling must take place, and each department or school of nursing needs access to a budget planning person who has the financial planning skills to assist with trend analysis and cohort-survival techniques. School budgets must be constructed around cost centers with decentralization of at least portions of the budget to smaller units, such as departments, which may be one cost center or be composed of a variety of cost centers.

Schools need to diversify, to search for new sources to generate revenue to offset salaries, such as faculty practice; training grants and research grants (with salary support and indirect cost recovery); joint appointments; contracts for the care of certain patient populations with such services as well baby clinics, senior citizen wellness clinics, and health department home visits; joint ventures with local businesses and industries, for example, offering work-study plans to their occupational health nurses and giving scholarship aid to employees' children; postpartum home visits provided by faculty to mother and baby for hospital patients who choose early discharge plans; proprietary interests in nursing homes and day care centers for infants and the elderly; and cooperating with a school of medicine to start a health maintenance organization as a full partner with medicine in the enterprise.

Schools and nursing service need to work with the marketing departments of many hospitals. Hospitals should begin advertising the quality of nursing care they provide—how many BSN nurses per patient they employ. As consumers are overwhelmed with cost-conscious advertising, an emphasis on quality will be appreciated and recognized.

Schools need to make hard decisions about the type and mix of faculty they need over the next ten years. Joint appointments and a tenure track and a clinical track will serve as a prelude to more involvement by nursing service in our educational mission.

Schools need to stop continuously revising curriculum and adopt a model that is cost-efficient. High costs used to be a badge of honor; now they are a competitive disadvantage. (Schools also need to decide with which schools they are competing, and then set tuition at a midpoint.)

Schools need to do more for less—to make use of the innovative approaches already discussed as we move toward "tighter" programs with a smaller number of regular faculty who are all doctorally prepared and other clinical faculty and preceptors who bring a rich blend of skills to our educational programs.

Alumni of schools of nursing must be better informed and the schools must reeducate them. Traditionally, nursing alumni have a poor record of donations. An enthusiastic development officer is a critical necessity for a school, and a wise dean cooperates fully in development activities.

Schools must examine cooperative agreements with other schools and with nursing services through which some costs may be shared and spread across a larger base, particularly in the areas of teaching and research.

Today, there is no room for dichotomy between nursing education and nursing service. As the old saying goes, "If we don't hang together, we most assuredly will hang separately"!

BIBLIOGRAPHY

American Association of Colleges of Nursing. *Economics of Higher Education.* Pub. Series 83, No. 1. Washington, D.C.: AACN, 1983.

Brown, E. L., and J. M. Lyons. *Analyzing the Cost of Baccalaureate Nursing Education.* New York: National League for Nursing, 1982.

Bureau of Health Professions. *Options for Financing Health Professions Clinical Education* (draft). Hyattsville, Md.: Health Resources Administration, March 1985.

Gonyea, M. A. *Analyzing and Constructing Cost.* New Directions for Institutional Research, No. 17. San Francisco: Jossey-Bass, 1978.

———. "Models for Faculty Development." Paper presented at the Fifth Annual Conference on Nursing Education, Albany, New York, September 22, 1983.

———. *Program Cost Analysis and Construction Methodology: Application for Nursing Education.* New York: National League for Nursing Research Division, August 1978.

Iglehart, J. K. "Difficult Times Ahead for Graduate Medical Education." Health Policy Report. *New England Journal of Medicine* (May 23, 1985): 1400–1404.

———. "Federal Support of Graduate Medical Education." Health Policy Report. *New England Journal of Medicine* (April 11, 1985): 1000–1004.

National League for Nursing. *Budget Management in Baccalaureate Nursing Programs.* New York: NLN, 1981.

Sloan, F. A., and J. Valvona. "Identifying the Cost of Graduate Medical Education." Paper presented at the Health Policy Symposium on Providing and Paying for Medical Education: Past, Present and Future, Vanderbilt University, Nashville, Tennessee, May 3–4, 1985.

BUILDING COHESION IN NURSING'S BODY POLITIC

MICHAEL M. HASH
Principal, Health Policy Alternatives
Washington, D.C.

The intent of this paper is to make several general points about the critical importance of nursing's role in the political process and how it may be strengthened, setting the context for more detailed examinations of the roles and opportunities for the nursing profession in the political arena. My experience in these matters comes from my observation of activities in Washington over the last 15 years and, more recently, my work with NLN and the American Nurses' Association. Much of this material is equally valid for other professional groups that seek to participate in and influence the political process at any level of government.

THE POLITICAL CLIMATE

To begin, some general observations about the political climate are in order. All of us are aware of the vast and rapid changes buffeting our increasingly interdependent world. One has only to look at the stresses and strains on the American economy arising from international competition to recognize that we are deeply affected by decisions made far from our borders. We are now also acutely aware of our finite resources and the kinds of painful choices those limitations impose. These developments have had a noticeable effect on our political process, and we need to be sensitive to these changes.

Most obvious from the perspective of the health care system has been the rise of competing claims for the resources that have been channeled into health services and research. What we are witnessing today are growing challenges to unlimited expansion of the health enterprise. The political process, to a large extent, acts as a broker for these competing claims on our national resources. A key factor in today's environment is that the struggle for resources is increasingly a zero-sum game—what one segment wins is at the expense of all other claimants.

In Washington and, indeed, in the state capitals, we are all experiencing the consequences of an economic pie that is not expanding as rapidly as the demands placed on it. We are now engaged in arguments about how to alter the size of the slices of the pie rather than how to bake a larger pie. For nursing and other health professions and providers, this has changed the outcome of political decisions and should cause us to reexamine our traditional approaches to advancing the goals of nursing.

Over the last five years, the decisions affecting national health policy have been driven almost exclusively by budgetary concerns. Interest in the substance of health programs and in questions about accessibility and quality of care has been eclipsed by an increasingly myopic view of the cost of health programs. Support for nursing initiatives and for nursing education and research has been set back by the relentless pressure of growing budget deficits.

A recent example of this is found in the ongoing saga of federal aid to nursing education. In most years, federal funds for nursing education represent the high-water mark for nursing lobbying efforts in Washington. Nursing organizations have developed strong alliances with the congressional committees that design these programs and the ones that appropriate money for them. The political leverage of nursing through its large numbers and its financial participation in political campaigns has been important to success in "bringing home the bacon."

In 1984, however, the president of the United States actually vetoed authorizing legislation to extend the Nurse Training Act, and in 1985, the Congress, preoccupied with budget deficits, is taking a very hard look at the future of these programs. Tough questions are being asked about the fairness of continuing support at previous years' levels when other programs—specifically those aiding the poor—are being cut back. Holding one's own in the present Washington environment is no mean feat.

Efforts to bring more focus and more clout to nursing research were given a big boost last year with congressional support for a National Institute for Nursing at the National Institutes of Health. Unfortunately, this proposal was also the victim of a presidential veto. This year, the outlook, again, is in doubt. Questions about financing a new institute when existing activities at NIH are being cut back again illustrate the kind of zero-sum game now being played in Washington.

These examples contain some important implications for the nursing profession as it seeks to advance its policies in this arena. Now, more than ever, nursing needs to broaden its public policy perspective—to look more aggressively for allies who might be willing to make common cause with nursing in return for aid on one or more of their objectives. As nursing has been absorbed with intraprofessional issues it has, to many on the outside, developed a somewhat parochial image. This has not served to promote the interests of nursing in Washington.

Now, with competition for resources more evident, the need for effective coalition building has never been more important. In politics, it's the numbers that often count the most: How many groups support a particular proposal? Where are they located? How many people will be benefited and in what ways? Coalitions help to provide the answers to these frequently asked questions.

The great risk is that the nursing profession may become too self-absorbed and too myopic as it concentrates on issues of professional identity. For example, no one in Congress is anxious to become involved in the issues surrounding the appropriate educational preparation for the registered nurse. From their point of view, this has become a "no-win" issue that should be resolved by the profession and at the state level. To the extent that segments of the profession seek to involve Congress in this issue, they will be eroding future political advantage at the federal level.

As nursing takes a broader view of public policy issues, it will be necessary to reexamine its Washington agenda. Historically, nursing has concentrated on federal aid for education, protection of the rights of nurses as employees, and coverage of nursing services under federal health financing programs—primarily Medicare and Medicaid. These have been critical issues for the profession, and much progress has been made in all of these areas. But the issues and priorities in Washington are changing. We need to take account of these changes and revise nursing's agenda accordingly.

We are all aware of the profound and rapid change in the way health care services are provided and paid for. Much of this revolution in health care is the result of actions taken by purchasers of services—government, insurers, employers, and individuals. New ways of paying for hospital care are dramatically lowering utilization and shifting the site of care. New delivery mechanisms are springing up like mushrooms—overnight. The growing supply of physicians and excess capacity in the hospital sector is fueling competition for patients and making providers more entrepreneurial in their professional behavior.

To a large degree, this has been the intended result of recent government policy to promote more competition in the delivery system as a means of containing health care costs. It seems to be working—at least in the short run. All the statistical measures of both cost and use are declining. What we are just beginning to learn is the cost of this success in terms of accessibility and quality of services and its impact on the health professions—including nursing.

PRIORITIES FOR NURSING

These changes lead us to take a fresh look at the nursing political agenda. What follows are some of my ideas about the priorities for nursing organizations in this new environment. The driving force behind federal health policy is to contain costs through the market power of a large buyer. I believe that nursing organizations should have a seat at the table when policy decisions are made about how Medicare pays for care. In the past, nursing has not given a great deal of attention to these issues.

In order to participate, nursing organizations must develop policies concerning these payment methodologies. More specifically, Medicare's prospective payment system, only recently implemented, is facing several serious challenges:

1. How to pay for the clinical education of health professionals.
2. How to measure the severity of illness of patients classified in the same diagnostic category.
3. How to finance the costs of care for the indigent.
4. How to pay for capital and new technology costs.

The nursing profession has a vital stake in the outcome of these policy debates, and, more important, has a contribution to make. Nurses certainly know something about the needs for nursing clinical education—not just in the hospital, but also in the ambulatory and managed care settings. Nurses are working on research to measure and analyze the costs of nursing care through various patient classification systems. Nurses have some experience with cost-effective models of providing care to those without financial resources. And, nurses ought to be thinking about the implications of a capital payment policy on nursing employment.

These are the health policy issues that will be debated in Washington over the next several years. The nursing profession should be a full participant in these debates, and steps have already been taken to prepare for that role.

Another issue that deserves high priority in the nursing profession is the measurement and validation of quality. The greatest risk that accompanies the moves to a more competitive and price-conscious health delivery system is the potential for compromises in the quality of patient care. As we all recognize, the financial incentive under many of the new payment arrangements is to underserve. Nurses are uniquely qualified to monitor quality and to help develop the tools necessary to assess quality in every setting. There is growing interest in this area at the federal level, among some physician organizations, and among consumers. Nurses can increase their visibility by stepping up their public support for quality-assurance mechanisms and through research to improve these functions. Nurses should continue their identification with quality-of-care issues in the health policy debates at every level.

BUILDING COHESION

In closing, I would like to emphasize a few points that can contribute to greater consensus within the profession on the importance of taking these issues on.

First, there needs to be more communication about what the critical public policy issues are. We need to make sure that the various nursing constituencies are knowledgeable about these issues and are committed to advancing nursing concerns that are relevant.

Second, there needs to be a concerted effort by nursing organizations to pull together resources from the profession to draw on their expertise in the development of policy positions that can be applied to these issues. This will not be easy, but it is clear that you can't come to the table unless you have a responsible position to advocate.

Third, there is a need to strengthen nursing's political bases. Public displays of divisiveness incur substantial political costs. The effectiveness of the profession in influencing the debates on health policy is compromised when there is evidence from the outside of fragmentation. In many respects, one of the most serious issues facing the profession (and other professions, as well) is the tendency for today's issues to divide. We need to find more effective ways of managing conflicts and resolving opposing points of view. Participation in the political process means building consensus. If nursing cannot accomplish this within its own ranks, it is not likely that it will enjoy much success in the larger arena of national health policy.

NURSING'S NATIONAL POLITICAL AGENDA

HAZEL W. JOHNSON-BROWN, PhD, RN
Director, Division of Governmental Affairs
American Nurses' Association
Washington, D.C.

The legislative and political agendas of the American Nurses' Association (ANA) have remained consistent over the past ten years. In that time, however, the legislative agenda has expanded; we have entered the regulatory arena with greater depth and knowledge, and we have increased our political savvy on the local, state, and national levels. Moreover, our strategies and tactics are changing. We are more vigorous and tenacious in the pursuit of our goals. ANA has moved beyond the era of narrow vision to wider focus on issues of the nation's health and well-being, such as the environment, discrimination and taxation in life and health insurance, organ transplantation and its attendant ethical issues, "Baby Doe" legislation and regulation, product liability, and funding for health care in developing countries.

During the past few years, we have seen a rapid rearrangement of the political and economic landscape. The milieu we are working in today is vastly different from the one that existed just a decade or even five years ago. Not too long ago, the emphasis in Congress was on new programs to meet social and health needs of various segments of the population and funding to foster innovations in health care. Today, the emphasis is on deficit reduction, cost cutting, deregulation, transfer of responsibility for social and health programs to states or the private sector, the threatened bankruptcy of the Medicare trust fund, severe reductions or elimination of federally funded health programs, and intense competition for the health dollar.

The federal government is moving in unprecedented ways in its efforts to cut the budget. Formerly sacrosanct areas such as Social Security and Medicare are being cut. Prospective payment and DRGs are reducing federal Medicare payments to hospitals. A freeze has been placed on physicians' fees under Medicare.

These actions have led ANA to give even more consideration to developing the political astuteness and acumen of its membership. To become politically savvy, it is important to build on the solid foundation of a national nursing agenda.

NATIONAL NURSING AGENDA

ANA developed the national nursing agenda in 1983 as part of a political education and action program conducted prior to the 1984 elections. The agenda addresses the broad range of nursing's concerns, outlining ANA's priorities in the following areas:

- Access to care
- Financing health care
- Funding basic needs
- Funding nursing education and nursing research
- Human rights
- Economic and general welfare of nurses
- Health hazards

Access to care in the national nursing agenda means working to assure access to quality health care services, especially for vulnerable populations such as children, the disadvantaged, and the elderly, and to assure access to nursing services. Under this heading, ANA supports such efforts as funding for maternal and child health; immunization and school health programs; access to long-term care services without excessive emotional and financial burdens on families; development or expansion of out-of-institution services, such as home health and community-based nursing services; and legislation to provide direct access to services offered by nurses.

ANA is concerned with *financing health care* to assure that the federal government maintains an appropriate role in determining the nature and quality of basic health care services and to assure that the federal government continues to work in collaboration with state and local governments to provide a stable source of funding to meet health care needs.

194

Under this heading would come legislation that removes barriers to the financing of nursing services and legislation that supports professional review of health care services of all health professionals for appropriateness and quality.

Funding basic needs means assuring a national policy and federal programs that meet fundamental needs of individuals for housing, food, education, and a safe environment—the basics whose lack jeopardizes good health. This agenda item refers to nursing support for such efforts as federal funding for the Women, Infants, and Children (WIC) food program.

Funding nursing education and nursing research refers to promotion of continued funding for nursing education, especially graduate education, designed to enhance the quality of patient care and the cost-effectiveness of health care delivery, and for legislation to establish a highly visible entity at the national level that focuses on nursing care research. Legislation passed Congress in fall 1984 to reauthorize the Nurse Training Act and to establish a National Institute of Nursing within the National Institutes of Health. Both were vetoed by the President, but were reintroduced in the House and approved by the Energy and Commerce health subcommittee in spring 1985. On May 22, 1985, the full Energy and Commerce Committee approved a three-year reauthorization of the Nurse Training Act. However, the committee rejected the recommendation of the health subcommittee to approve funding for 1986 at the level of $58.8 million. Instead, the committee voted 22 to 20 to freeze funding at the 1985 appropriations level of $50.3 million. The bill provides for a 5 percent increase in funding for 1987 and in 1988.

Human rights encompasses the drive for constitutional equality for women, civil rights, and voting rights. One measure that ANA pushed under this heading was the recognition of Martin Luther King's birthday as a national holiday. That is now a reality.

Economic and general welfare of nurses refers to legislation to protect the rights of nurses to organize and bargain collectively, enforcement of laws to protect the health and safety of nurses in their employment settings, and the elimination of sex-based discrimination in pensions, Social Security, insurance, and wages.

Pay equity continues to be a major issue in the women's economic agenda. Several bills have been introduced in Congress in 1985 that address various aspects of the pay equity issue. In the House, Representative Mary Rose Oakar (D–Ohio) introduced H.R.27, calling for a federal pay equity study, and H.R.375, dealing with pay equity enforcement in federal agencies. Rep. Olympia Snowe (R–Maine) introduced H.R.2472, which calls for a study of a federal agency under legislative control, such as the Library of Congress. In the Senate, Senators Daniel Evans (R–Washington) and Alan Cranston (R–California) have introduced S.519, which calls for a study of pay systems in the executive branch.

The Oakar Bill, H.R.27, has received the greatest attention and appears to have the best chance for passage. It is identical to a previous bill introduced by Rep. Oakar, which passed the House by a wide margin, 413 to 6, on June 28, 1984. Despite efforts by Sen. Cranston, however, it failed to clear the Senate. ANA has been actively supporting Rep. Oakar's efforts. We have testified at hearings held on the bill and have been working with the National Committee on Pay Equity to get organizational endorsements for the bill.

Health hazards as an agenda item entails support for the Clean Air Act, positive government action to prevent nuclear war, and programs for the protection of the environment and the public health.

Clearly nursing's concerns encompass a kaleidoscope of issues, but all are focused on better health care for all Americans and a more prominent role for nursing in achieving that goal.

LEGISLATIVE ISSUES

Major ANA legislative priorities include federal support for nursing education, particularly graduate education, legislation to foster the establishment of community nursing services, a National Institute of Nursing, and Federal Trade Commission (FTC) reauthorization.

Community Nursing Centers Act

The Community Nursing Centers legislation is a good illustration of how our tactics are changing. Community Nursing Centers legislation was introduced in the 98th Congress as the result of an ANA initiative. The idea for such a bill was and is a good one but because of several provisions in the legislation, it proved not to be politically viable. We must bear in mind that all elected officials, whether president or city council members, are faced with a multitude of constraints as a direct result of the positions they hold. They must contend as well with the added dimension of politics. And in today's political environment, especially at the federal level, the single largest issue is the deficit which continues to eclipse all other issues. Consequently, very few representatives are anxious to expand the federal government's fiscal role in any social program, especially health care.

ANA has therefore restructured its proposal to provide for a prospective funding mechanism for the provision of organized nursing services in a community setting—both to meet the demand for such services and to give recognition to nurses as primary health care providers. ANA is now proposing that the Medicare program "rebundle" existing ambulatory benefits into a package that health care consumers may utilize, to be provided by the most cost-effective providers, namely, nurses. The title of the proposal has been changed from "Community Nursing Centers," which implied the creation of physical entities, to "Community Nursing Services," which focuses on the services provided rather than the creation of institutions. By offering Congress a more cost-effective delivery system, we hope to garner additional support for both the proposal and the profession, while simultaneously demonstrating our concern for the need to reduce federal outlays for the costs of health care delivery.

Federal Trade Commission

The Federal Trade Commission issue was largely dormant in 1984, which meant that the FTC retained its antitrust jurisdiction over the health professions. Some groups, notably the medical profession, have been trying to remove the professions from FTC oversight. ANA has worked to retain that jurisdiction in the interests of freer competition among health care providers and the right of consumers to choose whichever legally qualified health care provider they wish.

In spring 1985, both the House Energy and Commerce Committee and the Senate Commerce Committee approved legislation to reauthorize the FTC, which has a good chance to pass. Many of the decisions regarding the jurisdiction of the FTC over the professions may be decided instead in the courts.

Nurse Training Act

The Reagan Administration's attitude toward the Nurse Training Act reflects the shortsightedness that characterizes its general approach to funding for health programs. Their argument is that there are enough nurses. Although this argument may perhaps be made, the point is that the nursing organizations have revised the Nurse Training Act in light of changing needs. Whereas formerly it focused on the shortage of nurses and on increasing their numbers, that is not the purpose of federal aid to nursing education today. Today the purpose is to meet the great need for nurses with advanced preparation to serve as nursing administrators, nursing educators, clinical specialists, nurse practitioners, and researchers. The Administration either does not understand or ignores that change in focus. Moreover, the emphasis on deficit reduction makes aid to nursing education and to other health professions highly vulnerable today.

As to the question of whether or not the shortage is over, I would point out that projections for the year 2000 indicate a supply of full-time equivalent RNs at just over 1.7 million, with a projected requirement of nearly 1.8 million full-time equivalent RNs. This forecast suggests that a modest shortage of RNs may persist over time. ANA's recently completed environmental assessment also indicates that changes in practice and demand will require an increasing proportion of registered nurses to achieve higher levels of education in the future.

National Institute of Nursing

Efforts to reduce the deficit also affect the push for a National Institute of Nursing. The Administration requested a cut in National Institutes of Health grants from the approximately 6,600 provided for in the appropriations bill to 5,000. However, in early June 1985, the Senate budget resolution raised the number of grants again to 6,000.

Although we do not actually have a nursing institute in place, nursing has gained much ground toward that goal in a relatively short time. Legislation creating the nursing institute actually passed both houses of Congress, only to be vetoed by President Reagan in October 1984. On May 15, 1985, the House Energy and Commerce Committee approved a one-year reauthorization of NIH, which included a provision for the establishment of a National Institute of Nursing. The substance of the legislation is identical to the bill passed in 1984.

Both the Public Health Service and NIH have conducted studies of the role of nursing research and nursing researchers in the federal government. Both of those reports, along with the earlier study from the Institute of Medicine, called for a stronger focus for nursing research.[1] A Center for Nursing Research has now been established within the Division of Nursing of the Bureau of Health Professions, Health Resources and Services Administration. While this is a step in the right direction, ANA is still committed to an institute, which we believe is essential to place nursing research within the mainstream of biomedical research.

NURSING'S POLITICAL ACTIVITY

Nurses are becoming more politically sophisticated, better able to deal with today's competitive political and economic environment. ANA's "Nurses: VIP Project"—standing for "nurses visible in politics"—was aimed at political education of nurses and building nursing's political clout. Four workshops were held in major cities with top representatives from both political parties. Recently, ANA played a prominent role in "Debriefing '84," a conference designed to analyze women's role in the recent elections and

---

[1] Janet C. Gornick and Lawrence Lewin, Lewin and Associates, *Assessment of the Organizational Locus of the Public Health Service Nursing Research Activities* (Washington, D.C.: Office of Health Planning Evaluation, U.S. Public Health Service, September 7, 1984); NIH Task Force on Nursing Research, *Report to the Director* (Bethesda, Md.: National Institutes of Health, December 1984); and Institute of Medicine, Division of Health Care Services, *Nursing and Nursing Education: Public Policies and Private Actions* (Washington, D.C.: National Academy Press, 1983).

assess the role of women in political life today. It generated a great deal of excitement in the political community, particularly because it was one of the few occasions when Republican and Democratic women got together to share information and experiences. It included female politicians from both the national and state scenes.

To further political education and action, ANA today has a network of congressional district coordinators in 326 congressional districts. A workbook is being prepared to guide their activities. Forty-one states have political action committees (PACs). A PAC survey has been produced and sent to state nurses' associations and to PACs to provide information on ways in which the development of state PACs can be assisted. ANA is also beginning to gear up for the 1986 congressional elections, with preliminary targeting of key races.

There is no doubt that legislators are more aware of nursing because of this political activity. Fully 88 percent of the candidates endorsed by the Nurses' Coalition for Action in Politics were elected in the 1984 elections. Nurses have captured the attention of policymakers.

AGENDA FOR THE FUTURE

Competition in health care, accessibility of services, and cost are the health care issues of today and of the future.

National health care expenditures have increased from $41.7 billion a year in 1965 to $355.5 billion per year in 1983. These skyrocketing costs have finally brought a change in congressional attitudes.

The American Hospital Association's *National Hospital Panel Survey*, whose reports are issued monthly, reported 1.5 million fewer patients were admitted to hospitals in 1984 than in 1983. Hospital occupancy dropped to 66.6 percent, the lowest it has been since the AHA began conducting the survey in 1963. It is interesting to note that there was an increase of about 1 million lower-cost outpatient visits during the same period. The survey also found shorter patient stays in hospitals—an average of 6.7 days in 1984, a 5.1 percent decrease from the average 7-day stay in 1983. Hospitals adjusted to this declining occupancy by eliminating about 11,000 beds in 1984, the first time the number of beds have declined for a full calendar year since AHA began keeping records. Hospitals also were employing about 73,000 fewer people in 1984, a drop of 2.3 percent from 1983.

These figures indicate a dramatic change in the health care picture. We are seeing a change toward something nursing has been recommending for a long time—a reduction in costly institutionalization and greater use of more cost-effective, ambulatory home care and community services, with more open competition to permit nurses to practice at their full potential.

The national nursing agenda is clear. It has not changed. We are adapting to a new milieu—one that can be threatening, but one that holds challenge and opportunity for nursing. In a very real sense, nursing is at the threshold of a new beginning. We are beginning to use all our talents.

Nursing's national agenda will continue to support goals to foster better health care for the people of this country:

- Continued federal support for nursing education to prepare nurses to function effectively in today's highly technological, highly competitive environment—to provide quality nursing services at reasonable cost in a wide variety of settings.

- Legislation that will assure access to health care for those who now are being squeezed out, such as poor women and children.

- Action to achieve a greater focus in the federal government on nursing, its contributions, and its potential contributions to health care.

- Support for actions that will open up more opportunities for nursing and prevention of actions that would militate against expansion of nursing services, such as the elimination of FTC jurisdiction over the health professions.

- Support for equal rights and pay equity that will assure women full equality and just remuneration for their work.

Nursing cannot be content to wait and expect someone else to accomplish the job of assuring excellence in health care. Nursing cannot be content to continue to play a secondary role in the health care delivery system. We must explore new and innovative ways to deliver services to those needing health treatment, education, and rehabilitation. We must support the efforts of our colleagues, nurses who organize to provide new modes of delivery of services in a community. Nursing must forge stronger links between the acute-care facility and posthospitalization community services. Nursing must gain and strengthen the leadership in the delivery of health services in nursing homes.

The American Nurses' Association will continue to educate the public, legislators, and consumers about the services nurses provide and will provide in the future. Each of the 1.7 million registered nurses is accountable for nursing practice. We must provide a high-quality service based on established standards of nursing practice and the Nurses' Code of professional ethics. Each nurse must understand the political domain and his or her responsibility in it.

Nursing has the political power to move the national nursing agenda forward. Nurses must clearly understand that as a collective we have a formidable power base. We must continue to educate ourselves in the collective use of that power. We need to truly heed the motto of the three musketeers—"All for one, and one for all." We have the knowledge, we have the power; we need the good sense to use it well and to use it now!

THE GREAT SHIFT: POLITICS AT THE STATE LEVEL

BETTY SKAGGS, PhD, RN
Director of Learning Center
School of Nursing
University of Texas at Austin

There has been a definite shift in recent years from politics operating at the national level to politics operating at the state level. We, the participants, are becoming increasingly sophisticated in playing the state political game, and we are playing it more actively and more astutely. We have learned from experience that we need strong participation in governmental processes at the state level if we are going to influence nursing practice and, ultimately, the health care of citizens.

At the state level, departments of health, departments of human resources, and other similar administrative agencies regulate many facets of nursing practice as well as the settings in which nursing care is delivered. Thus, nursing has learned, and learned well, that significant decisions affecting health care are made at the state level and that nursing must actively monitor the activities of state agencies.

For example, in one state familiar to the author, there have been numerous successful attempts to license allied health personnel, such as emergency medical technicians and respiratory therapists. In most instances, the practice defined for the allied health professional being licensed overlaps the practice of nursing and, if implemented, the legislation would represent a significant encroachment on the current scope of the practice of nursing. Therefore, nursing has had to educate bureaucrats, legislators, and lobbyists about the effects the proposed licensing bill

201

would have on the current practice of nursing. To date, we have been successful in amending both statutes and rules and regulations of these newly licensed or certified disciplines to protect the license and practice of nurses in this state.

Home health agencies offer another example of the nursing profession's work at the state level. The home health industry's strategy to contain competition in this rapidly growing industry included a licensing bill. In addition to regulating home health agencies, however, this bill would have required any nurse who practiced in a home setting to be licensed as a home health agency! If nursing had been regulated by this statute, then a school nurse who made periodic home visits to meet with the parents of a troubled child would have needed an additional license. The state nursing lobby was able to assure that nursing was exempt from this state regulatory body, preserving the integrity of the nursing board. Needless to say, a strong nurse lobby on the state level was vital to successful negotiations.

These illustrations are examples of reactive involvement on the part of nursing. We were responding to an immediate threat to our professional domain. Nursing, however, is assuming an active stance as well. The profession must be active in posing solutions to problems, not only in opposing the solutions of other groups. For example, the profession has joined (and even called together) coalitions to design resolutions to issues such as "Baby Doe" legislation, seat-belt regulations, clean air acts, and mandatory motorcycle helmet laws. In addition, in Texas, the governor appoints interim committees composed of legislators, community leaders, and experts in areas of concern to study selected issues. These committees formulate legislation to be introduced in the next session. Having established the professional nursing association as a source of consistent and dependable input, nurses have earned appointments to these prestigious committees. These mechanisms have proven to be effective methods of active participation in the health planning and in the decision-making processes at the state level.

The growth and maturity of the nursing profession, then, has led us to search for more effective ways to influence the health care system—to improve the quality and availability of health care. One logical avenue is political activity, especially state-level politics.

RESPONDING TO CHANGES

In addition to readiness on the part of the profession, the move to involvement at the state level was facilitated by certain social and political phenomena. One facilitator was the women's movement. Nursing, composed of approximately 97 percent women, has benefited greatly from the political involvement espoused by leaders of the women's movement.

In addition, many issues, such as child care for working mothers and women's health needs, translated directly from the women's movement to nursing arenas—and vice versa. In both nursing and the women's movement, political involvement seemed to enjoy parallel growth.

Furthermore, the nursing profession and the health care industry were adapting to societal changes described by Naisbett in *Megatrends*.[1] That is, shifts such as those from an industrial to an information society, from forced technology to "high tech/high touch," from institutional help to self-help, and from hierarchies to networking systems of organization, further reinforced nursing's unique contribution to the health care industry.

Finally, the political philosophy of the Reagan Administration presented new rules by which states would play. These new rules meant that the states would have more responsibility and accountability in developing and executing the various programs that over the past couple of decades had been under the control of the national government. This phenomena brought to light many new problems. State health plans and priorities had to be designed. In addition, innovative solutions were sought. In the flurry of activity, opportunities for new players became apparent. Perhaps most important, there was an excitement and a sense of urgency on the part of nursing to be involved in these activities. And nursing was ready to accept the challenge! We have learned the rules of the game. We have learned to create "win-win" situations through compromise. We have learned that our political enemies are not enemies—that even though we disagree on one issue, we will lobby together on the next issue. We know the art of negotiation. And, finally, we have learned how to expand our influence by not waiting for power to be given to us! We know what power is and how to use it.

USING POLITICAL POWER

We know that *expert* power (derived from knowledge), or the power base we use when we write letters and lobby our legislators, is important but not very effective. We have learned that we must work from stronger power bases. For example, more influential individuals work from a *legitimate* power base (derived from position). Too often nurses have seen individuals, such as physicians with greater legitimate power consulted for answers to nursing questions.

Realizing that nursing must develop its legitimate power base, nurses have gained prestigious positions, as members of school boards, city councils, hospital boards, and state legislatures. As a result, many nurses have established legitimate power and are recognized as community and

---

[1] John Naisbitt, *Megatrends: Ten New Directions Transforming Our Lives* (New York: Warner Books, 1982).

state leaders—simply by virtue of positions they have attained in the community. Legitimate power, coupled with a well-established expert power base, enables nurses to work more effectively in political arenas.

In addition, nursing has learned to use a third and even more influential type of power—*referent* power or *mentor* power (power gained from associates). Today, the profession has learned to use coalition-building as a method of expanding the skills and influence of nursing by sharing contacts, skills, and influence. A good example of exploiting this power base occurred in Texas during the 1981 legislative session. We were dealing with the issue of physician supervision of primary care providers. A significant number of primary care providers in Texas operate employee health clinics in the gas and oil industry. By helping the gas and oil lobby to appreciate the financial impact this issue would have on their industry, we were able to obtain their support. Their advocacy on nursing's behalf assisted us in reaching a satisfactory outcome.

Finally, nursing has learned to use the most powerful of power bases—the power to *reward* and *punish*. Today, nursing's political action committees (PACs) are well established. Our ability to make sizable contributions and endorsements (the reward mechanisms) is growing. Likewise, our ability to organize as a voting block to remove an elected official (the punishment) is also gaining momentum. Campaign contributions of state PACs and Nurses' Coalition for Action in Politics (N-Cap), the political action arm of the American Nurses' Association, have soared over the past couple of years. At the conclusion of the 1985 election cycle, one state PAC saw 90 percent of its endorsed candidates elected. Today, many candidates seek nursing's endorsement.

BENEFITS OF STATE-LEVEL POLITICS

More and more nurses realize that politics at the state level involves more than lobbying legislators when an issue comes up. Instead, they are able to view politics as one more tool they must use in order to deliver quality nursing care. As Jordan has reported:

> Nurses' beliefs and standards for health care will not survive in the future if exercised *only* at the bedside of patients and clients. Nurses' beliefs about health care must be transferred, via politics, into the actual health care system if nursing is to exist in the twenty-first century as a necessary component of health care.[2]

---

[2] Clair Jordan, "The Powers of Political Activity," in *Power and Influence: A Source Book for Nurses*, ed. Kathleen R. Stevens (New York: John Wiley & Sons, 1983), 83.

Strong state-level programs provide several other benefits to state and national organizations. These include (1) providing a training ground for young nurses; (2) permitting experimentation and creative problem solving; (3) allowing different solutions to meet unique regional needs; (4) providing feelings of involvement at a level closer to the "grassroots"; and (5) creating a track record for state legislators who move on to national positions.

In closing, as one examines the impact the profession has had on the health care system as a result of its involvement in politics at the national and state levels, most would agree that both the new skills and the new arenas are welcome additions. The individual, the state and national organization, the profession, and the patients have benefited. We need only to keep up the good work!

BIBLIOGRAPHY

French, J. R. P., Jr., & B. Raven. "The Bases of Social Power." In *Studies in Social Power*, ed. D. Cartwright, 150–167. Ann Arbor, University of Michigan, 1959.

Kraemer, R. H., E. Crain, and W. E. Maxwell. *Understand Texas Politics*. St. Paul, Minn.: West Publishing Co., 1975.

Sanford, Nancy D. "Identification and Explanation of Strategies to Develop Power for Nursing." In *Power: Nursing's Challenge for Change*, 15–26. Kansas City, Mo.: American Nurses' Association.

FROM BEDSIDE TO WHITE HOUSE: THE LOCAL PERSPECTIVE

DIANA J. MASON, MSN, RN
Lecturer, Lienhard School of Nursing
Pace University
New York, New York

Nursing is being referred to in political circles as the sleeping giant. Both within and outside of the profession, nursing's political potential is being recognized and, with increasing frequency, felt. Certainly, nursing's influence is being felt at the national level, largely through the cooperative efforts of the National League for Nursing, the American Nurses' Association, and the American Association of Colleges of Nursing—the Tri-Council for Nursing in Washington, D.C. With the shift of some power to the states under the Reagan Administration's New Federalism, nursing has also recognized the importance of politics at the state level, and has increased its activities in this domain. The local level, however, has received relatively little attention as an arena for nursing's political activities; yet this is probably the most important area to focus on if the profession is to realize its full political potential and become a waking, rather than sleeping, giant.

IMPORTANCE OF THE LOCAL LEVEL

There are several reasons why the local level is so important to nursing's political development. The first reason requires reexamining our concept of politics. In *The Political Action Handbook for Nurses*, Talbott and I define politics as any influencing of the allocation of scarce resources.[1] We have expanded the usual purview of political acion to include four spheres of influence with which the nurse must be concerned. In addition to the government, the most accepted sphere for nurses' political activities, we have included the spheres of the workplace, professional organizations, and the community. Until nurses increase their effectiveness in all four spheres, the potential power of the nursing profession will not be fully realized.

Nowhere is interaction between these spheres greater than at the local level. That is where nurses live, work, and socialize. The networks and influence nurses develop in our own communities and places of work can have an enormous effect on the professional images we build, the development of health policy, and the way we practice.[2]

Second, what we do on the local level can receive state or national attention and set precedents for others. For example, nurses in the District of Columbia formed a coalition to secure passage of a local law that prohibits hospitals from discriminating against nonphysician providers who are seeking hospital practice privileges.[3] The law is the first of its kind in the United States and has national significance. Solomon points out that the vote of the American Medical Association's House of Delegates to "provide financial support to fight both expansive nurse practice acts and expanded clinical privileges for nonphysicians makes the D.C. situation a critical one to watch."[4] The efforts of the D.C. nurses are important to all of us because they set a precedent for what other nurses can be doing and how they can do it. Local political victories for nurses can thus serve as models for the rest of the profession and the nation.

Third, with the trend toward decentralization, the local community is taking on a greater role in determining how scarce resources are allocated. There is a multitude of issues involving resource allocation at the local level. For example, in the mid-1970s, New York City was faced with a fiscal crisis necessitating cuts in vital public services. What was once *the* model public health department in the nation was forced to cut back its nursing staff drastically. A 1983 study reported that health services to public school children had become glaringly deficient.[5] Since the city is now financially healthy, it has acted on the report by allocating several

---

[1] Diana J. Mason and Susan W. Talbott, "Introduction: A Framework for Political Action," in *The Political Action Handbook for Nurses: Changing the Workplace, Government, Organizations, and Community*, ed. Mason and Talbott (Menlo Park, Calif.: Addison-Wesley Publishing Co., 1985).

[2] Anne D. Frost, "Working Together: Local Community Action," in *The Political Action Handbook*.

[3] Elizabeth Calderon, "The Organization in Action: D.C. Nurses Work for Practice Privileges," in *The Political Action Handbook for Nurses*.

[4] Sally B. Solomon, "D.C. Regulatory Battle Proves Our Fight Is Far from Over," *Nursing & Health Care* 6 (May 1985): 242.

[5] *Rx for School Children: An Overview of School Health Programs in New York City and Recommendations for Change* (New York: Citizens Committee for Children of New York, October 1983).

million dollars to redevelop the school health program. Instead of restoring its professional nursing staff to pre-crisis levels, however, the city claimed that there were not enough nurses prepared at the baccalaureate level who were interested in school health and decided to use much of the money to hire non-nurse school health "liaisons" who would coordinate the students' health care.

The growing influence of local government on health policy raises a variety of issues involving the quality of health care. For example, my New York City councilwoman wrote a discharge planning bill requiring that every patient discharged from a city hospital be given written discharge instructions by the physician or "to whomever the physician delegated the responsibility." It was clear from the last phrase that nurses would be intimately involved in implementing such legislation, yet the councilwoman had never consulted with nurses on the provisions of the bill.

There are also many nonlegislative issues that involve the politics of bedside patient care. In every workplace, nurses should be involved in influencing allocation of the scarce resources of time, supplies and equipment, personnel, and money.[6] The extent of nurses' influence within the health care institution may determine whether a staff nurse wastes precious time trying to locate one of two electronic thermometers (one of which is seldom working) or one of two sphygmomanometers on a unit of 30 or more patients, while the medical department has the latest in high-technology, high-cost diagnostic equipment.

Similarly, do we yet have sufficient influence within the institution and community to gain consumer and administrative support for improving nurse-patient ratios on general medical-surgical floors? These ratios have remained essentially unchanged for the past 20 years, while the patients become progressively sicker; yesterday's intensive care patients are today's general patients. Nurses on these floors know that staffing ratios are often unsafe. In the meantime, some hospitals are acting on warnings that nursing staff must be cut to reduce costs under prospective payment. If directors of nursing do not compromise on quality of care issues, their jobs may be threatened.

Many broader health and social issues at the local level merit nursing's attention. For example, the numbers of homeless in our local communities continues to grow. As increasing numbers of women and children join their ranks, we must begin to ask ourselves some hard questions about social policy in our communities and take a leading role in developing workable solutions to such problems. To confine nursing's focus to direct nursing care undermines nursing's holistic philosophy and will limit the scope of our influence.

---

[6] Diana J. Mason, "The Politics of Patient Care," in *The Political Action Handbook for Nurses.*

Because of the variety of health care issues that are influenced at the local level, we need to ensure that the nursing perspective on health care is represented at this level of resource allocation.

A fourth reason why the local level is significant to nursing is that enhancing nursing's political power at the local level serves to increase the profession's power at all levels. Mauksch contends that the most effective way to make deliberate social change is to target significant local groups and work to change their norms for accepted and expected attitudes and behaviors.[7] The local level can thus be an enormously important training ground in politics for the grassroots nurse—the base of nursing's political potential. Neglecting this level may mean missing a crucial opportunity to develop the political savvy of many nurses while building a foundation for political activism throughout the profession.

Political action at the local level is thus the foundation for effective politics at all levels and spheres of influence. Indeed, we ought to be careful in compartmentalizing nursing's political activities into local, state, and national levels, because in doing so, the interactions among the levels tend to be missed, and local political action is often relegated to a back seat when it may be most important.

BUILDING A LOCAL POWER BASE

What can we do to develop our influence in our local communities? While there is much that can and is being done, I will focus on two strategies that can do much to further our political clout: building relationships and demonstrating our expertise to the public.

Building Relationships

First and foremost, nurses need to expand our web of relationships within our communities. There are three groups, in particular, that nurses should be cultivating: consumers, legislators, and the media.

Consumers. The health care consumer is a resource that has been left largely untapped by nursing. When nurses have worked with consumers, they have had significant successes. The D.C. nurses' victory in securing passage of the clinical privileges bill owed much of its success to broad-based support from consumer groups that were part of the nurses' coalition, including the American Association of Retired Persons, The National Consumers' League, the Gray Panthers, and the National Organization for Women.

---

[7] Hans. O. Mauksch, "Political Imperatives for Nursing in a 'Stereotyping' World," paper presented at the National League for Nursing Convention, San Antonio, Texas, June 3, 1985.

The elderly, in particular, are a powerful group in many communities and, as frequent consumers of health care, can be natural allies of nursing. Women's organizations are beginning to awaken to the problems and concerns of traditionally female professions, and in many communities these groups have extensive political connections. The business community also must be approached as a consumer of health care, particularly as employers face burgeoning health insurance costs. Since business leaders are often among the power brokers in a community, relationships with this group can open many doors to power and influence.

Legislators and Their Staff. Relationships with local legislators and their staff are important for reasons other than local legislation. It is commonly known that members of the New York City Council have relatively little formal power in comparison with the mayor. And yet, as community leaders they can influence many events and issues.

About a year after I moved to New York City, I learned some important lessons about political realities and the influence of local legislators. I had not yet personally met my city councilwoman when I saw her in the audience at a June community program on teenage pregnancy. After the program, I introduced myself as a nurse and constituent, and asked her about scheduling a luncheon appointment with myself and several nurse colleagues to discuss nursing and health care issues.

She immediately asked me exactly where I lived, including which side of the street my building was on. When I told her, she noted that I would not be in her district when redistricting took place in September.

(*Lesson 1: Unless you are a constituent or a powerful person in your own right within the community, the legislator need not be concerned about you; after all, legislators must represent their constituents.*)

"But I am now," I insisted. When I repeated that I wanted to have lunch with her, she responded, "I'm awfully busy right now. I have a primary race in September and am in the middle of campaigning." I told her that I didn't need much of her time and suggested we schedule a meeting in her office instead of lunch. "You don't understand," she said, "I'm running a campaign and am very busy right now." Finally, it occurred to me to offer to do something to help her in her campaign.

"We're leafletting a neighborhood on Saturday morning and can use help," she replied.

"I'd be happy to help," I said.

"Wonderful!" she responded immediately. "Now let's see when we can schedule that luncheon."

(*Lesson 2: If I don't get her elected, she won't be able to do much for me anyway.*)

I helped the councilwoman distribute campaign literature for two hours on Saturday morning and, in the process, learned much about her and the community. I also attended a fundraiser for her, where I met the mayor and other important public officials and community leaders. We had our luncheon, and I found out that although she was an ardent leader on feminist issues, she was virtually ignorant about nursing. My colleagues and I began a long-term process of educating her about modern nursing and gained her respect.

As a result, the councilwoman has asked us for feedback on a variety of health and social issues that have come before the City Council. As author of the discharge planning bill mentioned earlier, she asked us to review it and make recommendations for revision. She has been a guest speaker for a local Sigma Theta Tau chapter program on politics and devoted one of her monthly cable television shows to problems surrounding the practice of nurse practitioners in the city. She offered to mobilize the local women's groups to support an informational picket by the nurses of the city's hospitals. And when nurses at a private hospital in the city protested the chief administrator's acceptance of the resignation of their director of nursing, tendered because of a practice issue, the councilwoman contacted a colleague on the hospital's board of directors, and the director was reinstated. And all of this in return for two hours on a Saturday morning, a delicious lunch, and a $25 fundraiser!

Campaign support is welcomed by local candidates because their races rarely get the media attention and monetary support of state and national races. The executive director of the Texas Nurses' Association, describes the development of a local nurses' political action committee (PAC) that played a significant role in two elections that later influenced nursing practice.[8] The PAC helped to elect a new mayor, who went on to appoint the first nurse to the board of directors of the city's hospital. The PAC also was instrumental in the election of a new sheriff, who subsequently reinstated professional nurses as providers of health care to the city's prisoners, who were then being treated by technicians.

New York City nurses do not have a local PAC, so we are participating in local campaigns in other ways. Two strategies that have brought us to the attention of candidates and have significantly influenced elections are writing health policy statements for candidates and "Dear Nurse Colleague" letters. These letters describe the candidate's positions and accomplishments and ask for nurses' support of particular candidates. They are signed by a number of prominent nurses and sent to nurses on mailing lists purchased from nursing associations.

The ways to participate are endless. The important point (Lesson 3) is that *participating in campaigns goes a long way toward developing significant relationships with legislators.*

---

[8] Clair Jordan, "Local Government," in *The Political Action Handbook for Nurses.*

Media. Competition for media time can be fierce. Often "who you know" within the media is as important, if not more so, than the issue. Yet one group of nurses was able to develop media contacts, get publicity for their issues, and make a significant difference in a key election, all at one time.

The local nurses' association in Syracuse, New York, decided to sponsor a candidates' night for candidates in local, state, and congressional races in their community. They invited a popular local journalist to moderate the debates. Since he had urged all his local newspaper, radio, and television colleagues to cover the program, the event received impressive news coverage, including one television news show outlining the major issues of concern to the community's nurses. Subsequently, there have been several positive stories on nursing by the news media. The moderator was invited by a director of nursing at the candidates' night to spend a day at her hospital and, after doing so, wrote a wonderful story on nursing. As an additional bonus, the nurses were instrumental in unseating a state senator who, as chair of the Senate Insurance Committee, had blocked for several years the third-party reimbursement bill for nurses. The bill passed in a special session of the legislature held after the elections.

Demonstrating Expertise

Relationships with consumers, the media, and legislators can be used in many ways to further nursing's influence in the local community. These relationships will be easier to form and maintain when nurses demonstrate our expertise to these groups. There are several ways to do this.

First, *develop a network of nurse experts.* The local nurses' association in New York City is compiling such a network. These nurses will be available to present testimony at public hearings, speak on radio and television shows, and address consumer groups. Recognizing that nurses who are experts in a clinical specialty are not necessarily expert presenters, the association has discussed plans for a workshop on public speaking, handling an interview, preparing and presenting testimony, and other skills to enable these experts to communicate their expertise effectively.

In many communities, there are nurses who are leaders in the profession on the state and national level. Unfortunately, too many of these nurse leaders no longer see the local domain as significant once they have made it to the "major leagues." When this is the case, nurses in the local community can lose a significant role model and spokesperson. Certainly, such leaders are often too busy to regularly attend meetings of nursing groups or do much work on a nursing committee. However, they can and should be tapped to represent nursing to the community at large and to lend their knowledge and leadership skills to the nursing community in selected ways. Finding ways to use our nurse leaders effectively for specific, time-limited assistance on the local level can do much to further our expertise and influence in our own communities.

Second, *get nurse experts appointed* to hospital boards, city commissions and task forces, and other public and private policy groups. The Texas nurses were successful in getting a nurse appointed to a hospital board because of the PAC. My councilwoman has suggested another way to get a nurse appointed to every city health commission and task force: Get a list of the committees and identify those that do not have a nurse member; send a telegram to the mayor pointing out these deficiencies; and the following day call a press conference announcing the lack of nursing representation on city health committees.

Whatever the strategy, lobbying for nurse representation on health-related committees is essential. Besides the influence on health policy that these committees may have, they offer access to important networks and power brokers in the community and give nurses an important opportunity to demonstrate and share our expertise with the community.

CONCLUSION

There is much that can be done on the local level of nursing's political domain. Clearly, developing political clout and expertise on the local level will enable nursing to significantly influence local policy and practice issues. Such efforts will expand the foundation for nursing's political power from the bedside to the White House.

SEEKING CONCILIATION: STRATEGIES FOR CHANGE

PATRICIA WINSTEAD-FRY, PhD, RN
Professor and Head, Division of Nursing
New York University
School of Education, Health, Nursing, and Arts Professions
New York, New York

This paper discusses change at the most generic level of all: that of the self. Nurses today are suffering from both low self-esteem and a poor image projected to the consumer. We need to examine the changes we might make in our approach to ourselves and our work as nurses that would lead to conciliation. I have chosen the word *conciliation*, rather than *collaboration*, which, according to Webster's dictionary, can mean "consorting with the enemy" and "compromising." *Conciliation*, on the other hand, means "to win over." There are two groups, then, that we must win over: (1) nurses ourselves, and (2) consumers.

A SYSTEMS VIEW OF HEALTH CARE

Before focusing on the changes that need to be made in the interests of conciliation, I will present a picture of the health care system from the point of view of someone with both a practice and theoretical background in systems theory. A systems-oriented person, who tends to see the world as interacting, connected networks, sees health care as one aspect of life in American society. It interacts with all other corporate, economic, and political systems. Practitioners of health care, whether dieticians, physicians, occupational therapists, or nurses, bring unique professional roles and values that interact in complex ways. The locus of intersection of all four domains—the corporate, economic, and political with the health care industry—is the local workplace—a college, hospital, home care setting, or the like. Today, people feel anxious and upset in that local workplace because for the first time in nursing's history, all four domains are changing simultaneously.

In the first half of this century, no one really paid much attention to health care. People sought care when they were sick. World War II changed that; the production of marvelous new technologies and drugs escalated during and after the war years. Third-party payment, which began in Texas, quickly caught on nationally. At first, however, third-party payers behaved much more like members of the health care industry than members of the economic community. In the good old days, health care providers submitted bills and they paid! Until recently, corporate America paid little attention to health care. Then big corporations began to realize that 20 to 30 percent of their budgets went to pay insurance premiums for employees. They began to wonder what they were getting for their money. Most recently, corporate America has begun to run health care agencies for profit.

As costs escalated, third-party payers began to behave more like economists than philanthropists. In the last 25 years, health care has become a focus of political debate and regulation, culminating most recently in the advent of diagnosis related groups (DRGs). Thus, today, the intersection of the health care industry with the other corporate, economic, and political domains is even greater. As this intense interaction, which has created the medical-industrial complex, has increased, the area of the intersection—the local level—has also increased. There is at least twice as much energy and interaction in any nursing arena today than there was a few years ago. The increased interaction also creates new areas for interaction that never existed before where health care intersects with one or more other domains—for example, corporate health care and nursing's political economic activity.

As people who are also nurses, we react consciously and unconsciously to this intense interaction. Hospitals lay off nurses to cut costs, only to find postoperative infections and other problems associated with hospitalization increase. Nurses who see themselves as caretakers and patient educators are finding themselves in a bind because DRGs do not cover caring. Nurses with an entrepreneurial bent perceive the current environment as ripe for private practice, establishment of buinesses, and other autonomous roles. It is truly a time both for new visions and for discomfort—a time of crisis. Crises are valuable turning points; one can emerge from them in better or worse condition.

CHANGING NURSING

Strategies for changing one's self and emerging from crisis in a better condition vary from stress reduction techniques to meditation to psychotherapy. I would not presume to recommend a single strategy for as large a group as nurses. I will instead, offer a few ideas on navigating through the uncharted area of today's nursing world.

Predicting the Future

The first idea is about avoiding traps. Avoid people who predict the future with certainty. As the discipline of futurology developed, one of the first things futurists discovered is that every prediction about what the world would be like in 20 to 30 years, except for forecasts of technological advances, has been wrong. The year 1984 came and went, but Orwell's Big Brother did not come. We are indeed poor predictors of our psychological and social futures!

One reason most people make such consistent errors is the fascinating, illogical processes that psychologists have found to underly what most of us would consider logical decision making.[1] These processes—*chance, representativeness* (a shortcut the mind takes to decrease the complexity of problems), and *availability* (judging the likelihood of something happening by how easily one can recall similar things happening)—operate in all decisions. People generally overestimate the likelihood of an event occurring if they can construct a series of events leading up to it that seem realistic. Consider the following scenario in which a nurse looks at her future:

She forms a premise:	"I think the hospital will lay me off."
She reacts to the premise:	"I'll organize the staff and we will unionize."
She predicts how the hospital will react:	"The hospital management will fire all of us, but the unionized employees will stand by us."

Before you know it, the nurse is picturing herself picketing in a snow storm and dying melodramatically of pneumonia. By using availability and representativeness, she has created a situation that she perceives as having a high probability of happening. The reality may be totally different; the entire scenario falls apart if the hospital doesn't lay her off.

---

[1] Daniel Kahneman and Amos Taversky, *Judgement Under Uncertainty* (Cambridge: Cambridge University Press, 1979).

Kahneman and Taversky caution

> Even with enormous uncertainties, some courses of action are better than others. But you shouldn't be very confident of your choices. Actions that acknowledge a high degree of uncertainty are often very different from actions that don't. It's frightening to think that you might not know something, but more frightening to think that, by and large, the world is run by people who have faith that they know exactly what's going on.[2]

Beware of hospital administrators, nurses, and anyone else who says, "If nursing doesn't get its act together and do *XYZ*, nursing is doomed!" Extinction does not occur that easily.

The Doctor-Nurse Game

The second situation to examine carefully is the nurse's role in the doctor-nurse game. Historically, nurses have spent a lot of time identifying with physicians, rebelling against physicians, comparing ourselves to physicians, and, in general, being highly emotional about physicians. None of these reactions signify a healthy relationship. DRGs were intended to decrease escalating health costs by decreasing the physicians' ability to generate costs. Physicians are "on the ropes" in the face of this attack on their power base. DRGs dramatically reduce their decision-making power. Several medical journals have carried articles on the decreasing power of the physician and the doom this spells for quality health care.

This is a prime opportunity for nurses and others to secure a portion of the power in the health care system, but it will take assertive planning and execution. Nurses who really believe they are "handmaids of the physician" will not be able to move and will seek to maintain as much of the status quo as they can. This realignment of the power structure will lead to some turbulence within our ranks for a while.

Technology

A third issue nurses need to reflect upon very carefully as we navigate through these turbulent times is our relationship to technology. As Pepper has recently pointed out, technology replaces people with equipment that automates some skills and thinking processes.[3] It de-skills jobs and makes some jobs that used to be interesting dull. Indeed, in intensive care units

---

[2] *Ibid.*, 26.

[3] J. Mae Pepper, "Future Direction in Nursing," address presented at the Annual Alumni Day, School of Education, Health, Nursing, and Arts Professions, New York University, March 1985.

217

today, computers are taking over some of the monitoring jobs that were performed by nurses. It is probable that some if not all the monitoring skills we teach will be performed by robots and computers in the near future. Even nurses' traditional association with drug dispensing will change. Implantable pumps are on the drawing board that can be programmed to dispense the correct amount of medication at prescribed periods of time. Yet educators continue to worry that students are not getting enough experience in managing the elaborate technology of modern medicine. To the extent that we prepare students for this as a primary role, we are educating for unemployment. Nurses in practice who perceive their primary role as monitoring machines are in jeopardy of being either bored or unemployed.

These are difficult questions, but if nurses are to seek conciliation with ourselves in these trying, hopeful times, we must find answers that we can live with confidently and that lead to action.

WINNING OVER THE CONSUMER

The other group nurses need to conciliate, to win over, is the consumer. Words such as *patient* or *client* have strong symbolic meanings to nurses. I deliberately call these individuals *consumers*, because as physicians and health facilities begin to advertise and compete for the patient's dollars, patients and clients will indeed become consumers. Except in emergencies, they will purchase health care as they purchase cars, appliances, and other expensive commodities.

Consumers are very confused today about health and illness. The media broadcasts every research finding, no matter how trivial or unscientific. Every talk show host regularly discusses health and illness, focusing on whatever topic is current and marketable. The general public consequently has a great deal of information on illness and its ravages, on what is wrong with our institutions, on the various sides of the malpractice issue and other problems. However, much of this material is presented emotionally and out of context. The end result of this flood of information is that people are confused and hope to avoid contact with the health care system. A recent Gallup poll showed that 85 percent of the people questioned try a home remedy before seeking medical help.

This is not to suggest that the American people are not interested in their health. The large assortment of self-help books on everything from childbirth to "deathing" attests to the public's concern for its welfare. However, the goal seems to be maximum health with minimum involvement of the medical establishment. The maintenance of health, which is nursing's sphere of activity, would thus appear to be a very marketable commodity. If nurses were to go into the business of marketing health, what would we sell?

Defining "Health"

To answer this question, we need to know what we mean by the word *health*. Probably no word is batted about more, but its meaning is frequently unclear. Smith investigated the literature to develop definitions of the term, and her review led her to posit four models of health.[4] They are the clinical model, the role-performance model, the adaptive model, and the eudaimonistic model.

The *clinical model* of health is the medical model. Most people who go to a physician are suffering from signs or symptoms of disease. The physician treats the symptoms or signs, and when they disappear the person is said to be healthy. In this model, health is the absence of disease. Disease is caused by some malfunction of the body's biochemistry due to heredity, a failure of homeostatis, or to the intrusion of some foreign substance (viruses, chemicals, or microbes). To determine how sick someone is, the physician uses the concept of the statistical norm. There is a normal range for blood pressure, organ size, blood values, urine values, and so forth. The physician uses the medical history, the physical examination and the various laboratory and X-ray analyses to arrive at a clinical judgment. Once this judgment is reached, the appropriate physiochemical or surgical technique is prescribed. People are viewed within this model as a mechanistic combination of organs and systems, like a car, which can be manipulated by a competent practitioner to achieve health.

The *role-performance* model of health derives from sociology. In this model, the individual is seen as having many roles to perform, and illness is that which impedes the performance of the roles. This approach has a certain commonsense appeal. When people are asked to rate their health status, they base their ratings on the ability to get around and take part in the activities that they consider appropriate for their life. This is a minimal definition of health, however, because people can also fail at roles for reasons other than poor health, for example, because they do not have the skills to perform them or because they are not motivated to succeed. Moreover, some people fulfill complex roles even with illnesses that are considered serious within the clinical model of health.

The *adaptive* model is drawn from the writings of Rene Dubos. He views health as a condition of the whole person involved in fruitful and effective interaction with the social and physical environment. Disease is a breakdown of the ability to cope with the changing environment. According to Dubos, one can be free of disease but not healthy. Illness can be privation, such as lack of clean air, inadequate recreation, or poor education. There are two types of adaptation—biological and social—

---

[4] Judith Smith, *The Idea of Health* (New York: Columbia University Press, 1983).

and success in both is necessary for health. Dubos's work highlights the reality of change in life. Health, then, is the successful management of life's changing environment. Like Hippocrates, Dubos believes that the role of medicine is a healthy society as well as a healthy body.

The *eudaimonistic* model draws from the philosophies of Plato and Aristotle; its modern patron is Abraham Maslow. Health in this view is measuring up to one's highest aspirations, self-fulfillment or self-actualization. To be merely satisfied is not health in this model. To be healthy, one must be exuberantly alive and growing. This model replaces the mechanistic view of the individual with a holistic one.

The clinical model is in trouble with everyone from public policymakers to the medical profession. Carlson and Cunningham have gone as far as to state:

> There have been no significant improvements in the public's health in recent years except for a small decline in the incidence of heart disease, attributable in large measure to improved diet and more exercise. At the margin, medical care appears to have stopped making a difference. Medical care aids many individuals in restoring and maintaining their health, but significant improvements in the overall health levels of the population are not being achieved through its provision.[5]

It seems fair to conclude that the consumer is more interested in approaches to health resembling the adaptive and eudaimonistic models than the clinical model. Consumers want to stay well, play golf, and relate happily to others.

Strategies for Winning over Consumers

Although nurse practice acts vary, many talk about diagnosing potential health problems and patient education. The American Nurses' Association *Social Policy Statement* encourages nurses to enhance the health of individuals, families, and communities.[6] Clearly, health, conceived as adaptive and eudaimonistic, is our domain. What strategies might we use to bring consumers to perceive us in this manner?

Obviously, the first step is marketing that image. This is already a major priority of Sigma Theta Tau, the nursing honor society, and many local and state groups, so I will make only one comment: whether the consumer is in the intensive care unit or on the tennis court, the nurse's primary

---

[5] R. Carlson and R. Cunningham, *Future Directions in Health Care* (Cambridge: Cambridge University Press, 1978), p. xv.

[6] *Social Policy Statement* (Kansas City, Mo: American Nurses' Association, 1984).

goal is health. In ICUs nurses observe, treat, and act to keep a bad situation from getting worse—we work toward health. Consumers are admitted to hospitals for two reasons: technology and nursing care. We cannot take a surgical suite to a home, so the person is admitted to the hospital. The physician thinks the consumer has an aneurysm, so the individual is admitted for nursing care: observation, rest, and education. Although acuity is a great concern, health and well being are the goals of nursing care. This is the image of nursing that needs to be shown to consumers.

Another strategy is assertive explanation of the nurse's role, especially in hospitals. It is frustrating to hear a consumer thank the attending physician for saving his or her life, when the physician was not even in the hospital. It was the nurse who observed the patient in cardiac arrest, called the code, and began life-saving measures! If the consumer were a psychiatric patient, we would say he or she was hallucinating, but we are so used to this misperception among other patients that we are not even surprised. Primary nursing and the movement toward home health care will help heighten consumers' awareness of nurses' role and responsibilities.

Finally, we need nurses with the skills and the savvy to go into the business of maintaining a high level of health—Nurses who speak and write and sell products of their invention to consumers.

To summarize, we have given service to the nurse-patient relationship for years. To some extent this has been lip service. It is time to make the nurse-patient relationship a marketable, real commodity. We need only remember that every contact with a consumer is a political act.

POLITICAL IMPERATIVES FOR NURSING IN A STEREOTYPING WORLD

HANS O. MAUKSCH, PhD.
Adjunct Professor
University of Wisconsin, Milwaukee and Parkside
Professor Emeritus
University of Missouri–Columbia
and
JAMES D. CAMPBELL, PhD
Assistant Professor
University of Missouri–Columbia

Stereotypes about occupations vary in detail and force. The professions tend to have more visibly developed stereotypes and more strongly developed links between these perceptions and the public's judgment and expectations about the profession. For some occupations, stereotypes are primarily positive and advantageous, whereas negative stereotypes are the burden of others. Nursing exists in the midst of complex images that offer a mixed message of support and hindrance to the profession. To further the ends of a profession may require altering significant components of selected stereotypes. This requires political use of image management, public relations, collective psychology, and political alignments.

Specific problems for the aims of nursing are created by the fact that some of the most pervasive stereotypes about nurses are not only formidable obstacles to the acceptance of nursing as a serious, specialized profession, but these stereotypes are also viewed by the public as being "nice," flattering, and desirable. Many of the images of nursing are rooted

The study reported in this article was made possible by a grant from the W. K. Kellogg Foundation. This paper was presented at the NLN seventeenth biennial convention by Dr. Mauksch.

in deeply held stereotypes about females and are linked to the perception of women as generalists and nurturing figures who resort to "natural" talents when they do what they do. To change stereotypes based on negative perceptions is easier than to alter images that are perceived as primarily positive, loving, and supportive—when in fact they are patronizing, demeaning, and limiting.

The profound impact of stereotypes became dramatically clear during the conduct of an evaluation project of joint practice—the presumably collegial cooperation between nurse practitioners and physicians in primary care. Although the evaluation of joint practice, which focused on family care, examined many other questions, the importance of stereotypes and their impact on providers, clients, and institutions was always forcefully obvious.

STEREOTYPES IN JOINT PRACTICE

In rendering primary care, images of outcome and priorities influence the behavior of the providers and the judgments made by them and by patients. In observing joint practice teams, the researchers were able to identify a range of nursing and medical activities. The behaviors observed were frequently not the behaviors recorded by the providers. Even nurse practitioners who had formed strong opinions about the egalitarian attributes of team practice were found to place a higher value on medical activities than on nursing activities in their records and reports. The discrepancy between the actual behavior coded by the observers and the claims recorded by the providers expressed traditional socialization rather than professional beliefs.

The stereotype of patient care places much greater value on cure than on care. Furthermore, the preeminence of the medical model is partly due to the recognized inequality of power, partly due to the relationships between the genders, and partly due to the deference given by younger people to older ones. In addition, the nature of the employment contract and the structure of the practice setting frequently militated against a change in the traditional stereotype of the hierarchical arrangements between nurses and physicians.

The stereotype persists that whatever the physician does is more central to the ultimate goals of patient care than the activities of any other provider. One of the most important components of the comprehensive stereotypes that nursing must address is the perception that what nurses do falls within the medical domain and represents essentially the performance of delegated and transferred activities. A microanalysis of taped patient care encounters revealed that nurse practitioners do indeed perform activities that are distinct from those performed by physicians. Frequently, these may be identical activities, such as taking a history or doing physical assessment, yet the objectives of the activity and the use of the information varies between the two professions, as does the style of their performance. Since change of public images must start with the self-image of the group in question, it is important to note that nurse practitioners in almost all instances undervalued their activities as shown in charts and records. Many concentrated on activities that "would be of interest to the doctor."

To liberate the practicing nurse is not merely a sociopsychological necessity; it is a political imperative for initiating meaningful changes and breaking through this stereotype-based prison that keeps nursing from claiming its share of credit and respect. The prevailing image that the physician's activities are the measure of patient care is deeply rooted in the public's perception, the media, and the beliefs of the members of both professions. Some argue that this is a good enough reason to give up on cooperative arrangements between medicine and nursing—that the reality makes cooperation impossible. On the contrary, changes in images and perception will not occur if the issues are avoided and buried. The prevailing patterns can only be altered by strongly organized, well-documented, and politically sophisticated alterations of past stereotypes. The observations of teams that are functioning reasonably well, although few in number, support the optimistic expectation that, at least within these teams, past stereotypes do change and new insights and changed relationships will emerge. Such foci of change may have the potential to influence their environment and sustain a consistent pattern of change.

CHANGES ON THE HOME FRONT

These aims not only require patience. They require the acceptance of the challenge on two fronts: with the public and within the profession. An effective effort to clear the road ahead of obstructive stereotypes can occur only if the first battle is conducted on the home front, that is, changing the stereotypes that are affecting nursing itself. The first goal must be the development of pride and autonomy and the fostering of loyalty to other nurses. We observed that, in interviews, nurse practitioners were not always comfortable with claiming the importance of their own contribution to patient care. To believe that the substance of one's work is under one's own control and that it derives from the domain of one's own profession affects the feeling of worth, the posture of secure assertiveness, and the willingness to be counted.

A dramatic example of the consequence of stereotyped thinking could be observed in a number of joint practices in the upper Midwest. A number of physicians working closely with a nurse practitioner would tell us, as if it were a secret, "If I could get another physician to work with me instead of the nurse practitioner, I would say, 'No, thank you.' Working with the nurse practitioner, we give much better care. We complement each other. You understand, however, that I cannot let my colleagues know how I feel." In such settings, the nurse practitioners would frequently indicate that they knew they were respected and that they understood as well that the physician could not show it. The fact that such an arrangement has to be treated like a guilty secret is testimony to the power of stereotypical thinking, even though it also relates to other problems. We found that joint practice was a threat not only to the community of physicians but also to traditional nursing, primarily hospital staffs. Here we ran into the stereotype that a nurse ought to be supervised and that nurse practitioners were disturbing because they did not fit into a supervisory structure. This is quite a stereotype for a group that claims to be made up of individual professional practitioners!

We did find that egalitarian, collegial relationships within the joint practice team were more likely to emerge the farther the team was from either hospitals or other practicing physicians. One of the unfortunate by-products of the discomfort about joint practice and the conflict of images could be observed in the granting of attending privileges to nurse practitioners. While medical staffs generally had no problems with such arrangements, in a large number of the situations we observed, the nursing service department refused to grant attending privileges to nurse practitioners. In North Dakota and South Dakota, we found that many nurse practitioners resorted to licensure as physicians' assistants to bypass hospital nursing and to obtain hospital privileges through the medical staff. For some nurse practitioners, this was a difficult choice to make. Although the role of researcher requires the ability to look dispassionately at data, it was hard to avoid sadness and regret when observing such instances of professionals behaving so destructively toward their own profession.

LEARNING FROM OTHERS

There is another reason why responding to stereotypes must start at home. Objectives of professional development and emancipation may not only be serving professional purposes, but may be essential political tactics. A lesson can be learned from the many oppressed groups who have suffered throughout the history of the human race. Studies of blacks, Chicanos, and women have demonstrated forcefully that the most pernicious and destructive consequence of socialization into the oppressed status involves the formation of a damaged self-image. The negative messages about one's fellow victims infiltrates the self-image and results in the message that one cannot really trust one's own group and that one's peers cannot be very important. This tendency for self-destructive and self-devaluing feelings applies both to the view of self and to the entire oppressed group. Feelings of collective pride, of loyalty to the group, and a commitment to the well-being of the group are not likely to result from this kind of socialization.

History teaches us that oppressed groups develop a sense of assertiveness only after anger has been allowed to boil and bubble and the group closes ranks under the flag of protest and rebellion. Whether it is the cry that "Black is beautiful" or the feminist call for the power of sisterhood, the damage of negative images historically has required the application of noisy rhetoric and expressive action. Even those who may be repelled by the noise and by the lack of aesthetics should remember that history shows that corrective action may not be able to occur without causing a great deal of heat.

Although not central to our research questions, informal contact and some content from the formal interviews pointed to the frustration among nurses with the profession's preoccupation with differences and distinctions within its ranks. This emphasis occurs, many feel, at the expense of a commitment to unity and the pursuit of overriding common interests and goals. Purely on the basis of politics, without resorting to more important professional and personal considerations, the overriding need for the profession seems to be the fostering of a sense of loyalty to one another, a commitment to common goals, and a sense of pride.

Admittedly, this emancipation of the self-image has been a different challenge to various minority groups. It was a strategic advantage to the black community that it could, at least symbolically, isolate itself from the white world to work up the steam and create the symbols that were needed to initiate change. The women's movement found this tactical separation somewhat more difficult to translate into political action, and the family, at times, became either a battleground or neutralizing territory. Again, the call for sisterhood was an effort to create a rallying focus. The nature of patient care makes it even more difficult for nursing to declare its identity as separate from and not related to the function of other professions. Some nursing leaders call for a complete separation of nursing from medicine.[1] However, this does not seem to be a viable option in the majority of patient care settings, particularly in acute-care institutions. The belief in "nursing power" is an essential prerequisite for improving the sense of self-worth among nurses and for enhancing the political effectiveness of encounters by nurses with others, whether professionals or clients.

NURSING AND GENDER STEREOTYPES

Inextricably interwoven with these issues of nursing worth and nursing self-image is the stereotyped identification of the nurse with the female

---

[1] Martha E. Rogers, "Nursing: To Be or Not To Be," *Nursing Outlook* 20 (January 1972): 42–46.

gender. The stereotype of the nurse as a female has far-reaching implications in both obvious and subtle facets of the nurse's existence. The demeaning and sacrificial games played in patient care have been described as the doctor-nurse game.[2] They always involve the substitution of personal, stereotypically feminine techniques for professional relationships and thereby reinforce the survival of subordination and traditional images. This pattern may include more overt forms of sexually flavored approaches and it may involve the playing of games in which the rules favor the boys.

Much less obviously, gender stereotypes affect the role of the nurse by creating the expectation that the female is the generalist and the manager, whose competence emerges from natural talents rather than from learned skills. Studies of communication between nurses and physicians reveal the paucity of professional information that is permitted to flow from the nurse to the physician. This balance seems significantly improved in joint practice.

A much more subtle aspect of the gender stereotype is associated with the notion that when women are defined as expressing their natural needs and talents in their work, the rules of the marketplace can be reinterpreted. Since economic rewards must be less important to people who are doing what comes naturally, the rules of contract change. Although this stereotype still exists, it has, in fact, been significantly modified in the last ten years. It deserves mention, however, because its refutation still requires concerted action and surveillance.

In the various joint practice settings that were observed as part of the study, an entire range of accommodations was observed. The relationships between male physicians and female nurse practitioners ranged all the way from those only minimally different from traditional hierarchical structures, to arrangements in which there was not only a contract but a reality of continuous partnership and shared decision making. Not surprisingly, the more egalitarian relationships usually involved younger physicians. This finding offers some hope.

In some instances we felt that it was the nurse practitioner who maintained the traditional relationship despite the physician partner's willingness to go beyond this. Our experiences confirmed the consistency of a subtle semantic clue to the nature of the hierarchical relationship that prevailed in a joint practice. Normally, the nurse practitioner met first with the research team. If the nurse practitioner told us, "Doctor will be here in one hour," we would anticipate a traditional physician-nurse hierarchy. If she remarked, "The doctor will be here in one hour," the scenario would be more unpredictable and varied. The most collegial conditions could usually be expected when the nurse practitioner said, "Doctor Grove will be here in one hour."

---

[2] Leonard I. Stein, "The Doctor-Nurse Game," *Archives of General Psychiatry* 16 (June 1967): 699–703.

POLITICAL OPTIONS FOR NURSING

What political options are available to nursing in the light of existing conditions? Obviously, the two extremes are that nursing can respond by calling for a revolution or, conversely, that nursing can teach its novices to adjust to existing reality and let current conditions remain the norm. Neither of these two extremes are likely to be the choices of the profession.

Three further options remain. One of these addresses the change of images as a public relations campaign and essentially involves the selling of new perspectives. The second approach is directly aimed at the individuals who, either as co-workers or as members of the public are involved with nursing. This second approach seeks to convert. It seeks to change actual beliefs and perceptions. The third approach addresses the values and norms that govern the behavior of identifiable small groups, such as work environments or neighborhoods. It assumes that human beings see what they are expected to see and that they are sensitive in their attitudes and their behavior to what they believe to be expected of them.

There is a place for the public relations approach. This society is responsive to media messages. Although greater concern with the media and with monitoring of media messages may be a necessary political stance of nursing, it cannot be a sufficient one. The delicate nature of stereotypes and their deeply rooted persistence require a more pervasive approach. The effort to convert individuals seems much more appealing, but it is a slow and inefficient approach. It is made even more difficult if one admits that the opinions held by individuals are only partly rooted in their own personal belief system. For most people, stereotypes and images are shared with significant social groups from which the individual derives the cues and the approval for the views expressed and the attitudes proclaimed.

This realization leads us to the third approach, which derives its formulation from Myrdal's classic study of the "Negro in America."[3] In addition to its substantive information, this report contained one of the most effective models of planned social change. One of Myrdal's points involves the appreciation of the powerful force that perceived expectations have on individuals. Thus, the perceived norm in universities is that only research and publication count toward tenure and promotions and that teaching is not as important. In a brief study of six institutional tenure and promotion committees, the senior author found that no more than one-third of any committee interviewed actually voted their real conviction. When interviewed alone, the majority acknowledge that personally they

---

[3] Gunnar Myrdal, *An American Dilemma: The Negro Problem and Modern Democracy* (New York: Harper & Bros., 1944).

would have liked to give greater reward to teaching, but that they did not vote that way because they knew that the majority expected them to support the preference for publications. In every one of these institutions, the majority of the promotions and tenure committees perceived university administration as considering only publication records. Oddly enough, every one of the academic vice-presidents interviewed felt that the faculty promotions and tenure committees were too rigid about publication requirements and would have liked to see more recognition of teaching.

The reinforcing nature of perceived norms has a life of its own, and these norms are sometimes dramatically different from reality. To change the images about nursing may require not the change of individual views, but rather, it may be optimally addressed by changing the climate of perceptions, descriptions, and jokes that are tolerated and approved within the perceived norms. When it becomes acceptable for physicians to acknowledge their gratification with the team relationship, and when physicians silence a colleague who makes sexual innuendos about nurses as entertainment, changes will have taken place. When it is perceived as normal for nurses to take the lead in the discussion in a multiprofessional environment and to assert nursing's contribution as uniquely their own, changes will have taken place. When a hospital administrator or a director of nursing acknowledges the claims that derive from the nurse's specialization in given areas of practice, rather than sending the nurse to any possible corner of the institution, and when the hierarchy acknowledges the expertise of the practicing nurse as an autonomous characteristic of the profession, change will have taken place.

The lessons of the study of joint practice have reaffirmed the persistence of the image problems that have plagued nursing. Yet they have also shown a basis for hope and the potential of success through concerted action. To be successful, action must involve nurses themselves and draw on their commitment and their sense of loyalty to each other. It must also accept the fact that political success is not the result of merit, but rather the consequence of hard work, good organization, and sophisticated use of resources.

themes and images
for the future

NURSES AND PATIENTS TOGETHER: HEALING THE HEALTH CARE SYSTEM

MARGARET E. KUHN
National Convener
Gray Panthers
Philadelphia, Pennsylvania

There is much to say about our responsibilities in this age of tumult and terror. Tumult, because of two revolutions sweeping across the world—the demographic revolution bringing a totally new challenge, with more people living longer than ever before in human history; and the technological revolution radically changing the nature of work. While the demographic revolution is a triumph of public health, with improved sanitation and eradication of infectious diseases and epidemics, it collides with the technological revolution, which has brought the robotizing of work, automated assembly lines, and the wasting of the skills of two generations of older workers. Technology has improved life and prolonged it, but we need criteria to determine what technology is appropriate.

To complicate these revolutions, we see the ravages of racism, sexism, and ageism, which are pervasive social sicknesses rooted in our profit-centered, competitive, economic order. Both nurses and patients must be part of the liberating struggles to stamp out these social sicknesses. We know that the malaise of society affects the health and well-being of all of us.

Human survival, safety, and happiness demand cooperative efforts of patients and health professionals working together for the social changes essential for justice and peace. The healing of society and the healing of the health care system go hand in hand, but the healing is not without risks, setbacks, and controversy. These are inevitable but exhilarating when we experience them together. Our diagnosis must recognize the economic and social roots of poverty, economic oppression and exploitation, hunger, and homelessness, and how they affect health and well-being. In a society where the "bottom line" is a priority, segregated lifestyles and the stereotyping of people by race, sex, social class, and chronological age are enforced and perpetuated. New attitudes, mass education, and new cooperative ways of living and working are necessary to liberate ourselves and our society from racism, sexism, and ageism.

Nurses have had a significant part in the liberation of women. The autonomy of nurses, the development of new professional roles—the nurse practitioner, the nurse midwife, the geriatric nurse—are exciting and affirming. Nurses encourage the liberation of older women from the restrictions and stereotypes of ageism.

Our diagnosis of society must also recognize the malaise in the health system. It is privatized, individualistic, fragmented, specialized, class divided, overpriced, and committed to acute care, miraculous cures, drugs, and surgical interventions. It has grossly neglected chronic diseases and the prevention of disease and health promotion.

We must also check the race toward the corporatization of health care. Nurses and patients are becoming aware of the powerful influence of the American health empire, which links drug companies, manufacturers of hospital equipment, the insurance industry, and the developers of the artificial heart with hospitals and medical schools. Multinational conglomerates are growing in power and profitability. Humana and the American Health Institute, for example, are buying up nonprofit hospitals, nursing homes, and home care services. Aggregates of economic power generate big bucks! The goals? Efficiency, yes. Profits, of course! Who has access to the system? Who is admitted for care? Who is *not* admitted for care? Who is discharged? How effective is discharge planning? These are urgent matters for nurses and patients to explore together.

Under the prospective payment system and diagnosis related groups (DRGs), those patients who have some form of medical insurance, including hospital insurance, may be admitted. What we have noted to date about the discharge procedures makes us very anxious. We have observed the discharge of patients after the prescribed length of hospitalization, with temperatures and conditions far from stabilized. Undoubtedly there was abuse and inappropriate use of hospital care before, but the present corrective measures can lead to other abuses far more serious to the person and to society.

The corporatization of health care will make radical changes in the decision-making processes in hospitals and nursing homes. The physician's decision may well be outweighed by corporate economic policies and decisions made in a corporate head office miles away from the person who is sick and requiring care. It will establish, we predict, a three-tier range of care. The first tier will provide the affluent with everything they need and want. The second tier will meet most needs of the patients with health insurance. The third tier will give minimal care to the poor and the uninsured, who are lucky to be admitted to care.

Gray Panthers have made health care a priority for more than a decade. As our national Health Task Force studies the issue of health care for profit, we are deeply concerned about the people who will not be admitted to care—the tens of thousands of people of all ages who have no health insurance or health benefits provided by employers. We are concerned about the health of the unemployed. Our concern was reemphasized by the experience of serving for two years on a Mayor's commission for the study of health care in Philadelphia. Thirty commission members, assisted by eleven committees, probed every aspect of health care in the city, including all aspects of public health. When the report to the mayor was presented in June 1984 with 483 resolutions, the commission found that the largest factors influencing the health problems of Philadelphia were unemployment and poverty.

STRATEGY FOR HEALTH

The Gray Panther health strategy is to support and work for a national health care plan similar to what we have observed in Canada. Ten of us spent a week in Montreal in April 1985, studying in depth every aspect of the provincial health care system. We were free to interview all kinds of people in French and English. We walked through neighborhoods and the wards of hospitals and extended care facilities. We talked to nurses, physicians, and social workers, who work together as a team and who consider health care an intrinsic part of a comprehensive social welfare system that benefits every Canadian, regardless of income, age, occupation, residence. In our intensive interviews we found an absolute commitment to the health care system in Canada. The Canadians enacted their health care plan by securing provincial approval and adoption of provincial services.

Gray Panthers are now concentrating on a state-by-state strategy. In New York state and Massachusetts nonbinding resolutions have been introduced, calling for a referendum on a state system. Gray Panthers plan public education campaigns to stimulate voter interest and support. We hope that nurses' associations in these states will be a part of this voter education effort. Nurses and patients can be powerful allies in these state campaigns.

The Gray Panthers believe that the corporatization of health care, the present prospective payment system, and the growing instances of malpractice suits all work to create a climate in America that will make the Canadian system a viable and attractive system for us.

We have socialized medicine in the United States for every member of the armed forces, for veterans, and for members of Congress. If the services are right for them, why are we deprived of them? What are we waiting for? I have a vision of hospital acute care and other institutions becoming obsolete because they no longer serve the public interest. We cannot substitute "efficiency" and profitability for quality of care and compassion.

Gray Panthers have also been studying the workings of the hospital chains. Humana has developed the artificial heart and has received tremendous national publicity. Humana is buying up a number of hospitals in the Chicago area. We are told that there is a plan to build a medical school that Humana will run. Our plan is to recruit a small group of patient advocates who will monitor the care in these for-profit hospitals. We will be watching who is admitted and who is not admitted. We will be evaluating discharge procedures and plans. We will look at the interpretation of the Patient's Bill of Rights.

We realize that it will take persons who know the hospital system to observe these matters. Older nuns in several communities have talked with me about how they could help, and we need nurses' help in developing this plan to recruit cadres of older nurses, including nurses in nursing orders, to be the patients' advocates in four hospitals that are run for profit. With the data compiled by the nurses' advocates, we will have important material for stockholders' resolutions. Part of this plan is the purchase of hospital corporation stock and going to stockholders' meetings with resolutions that will not stop the corporatization of health care but that will sensitize and alert the industry.

Health care is a basic human right. It ought not to be, as it is today, just for those who can afford it. We believe that sooner or later the United States will be ready to adopt our own version of the Canadian health care system. The corporatization of health care will move us in this direction.

NEW MODELS OF CARE

Nurses are advocates and always have been. Nurses and patients have a system and the building of a coalition that would support the social and political changes necessary for universal care. Moving in that direction, I see some exciting new models of care: wellness centers, patterned after the marvelous holistic health care center of which I am a member in Philadelphia. Located in a Germantown Episcopal church, it is committed to care of the body, mind, and spirit and to the environment. It is a wonderful totality of compassion and concern.

236

The Gray Panthers are working with the holistic health center and the University of Pennsylvania School of Nursing in the design of "healthy blocks," using health as an organizing principle for reconstituting blighted, declining neighborhoods. The goal is holistic health for all the residents of the neighborhood—all the babies and children, all the working adults, the old people and the young people. "Health builders," who are neighbors, will be trained by the holistic center staff to be the health workers and health promoters. The holistic center provides the backup staff.

We also see health cooperatives, with services paid for cooperatively. We see teams of nurses developing the marvelous variety of services which they provide.

To summarize, we see nurses and Gray Panthers working together, buying shares of stock in health conglomerates. We see retired nuns monitoring health care for profit, gathering data to bring to stockholders' meetings, mingling economic perception with concern for justice and health.

It is a great vision, and Gray Panthers love the idea of working with nurses and learning from nurses. What are we waiting for?

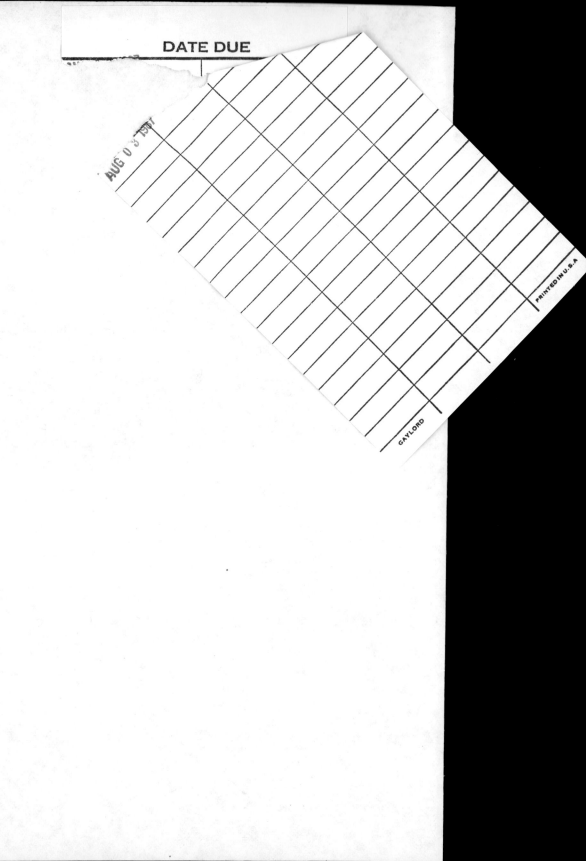